Nursing Care for Cancer Patients

Nursing Care for Cancer Patients

Editor

Qiuping Li

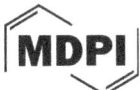

Basel • Beijing • Wuhan • Barcelona • Belgrade • Novi Sad • Cluj • Manchester

Editor
Qiuping Li
Wuxi School of Medicine
Jiangnan University
Wuxi
China

Editorial Office
MDPI
St. Alban-Anlage 66
4052 Basel, Switzerland

This is a reprint of articles from the Special Issue published online in the open access journal *Healthcare* (ISSN 2227-9032) (available at: www.mdpi.com/journal/healthcare/special_issues/68R0236YJA).

For citation purposes, cite each article independently as indicated on the article page online and as indicated below:

Lastname, A.A.; Lastname, B.B. Article Title. *Journal Name* **Year**, *Volume Number*, Page Range.

ISBN 978-3-0365-9896-3 (Hbk)
ISBN 978-3-0365-9895-6 (PDF)
doi.org/10.3390/books978-3-0365-9895-6

© 2024 by the authors. Articles in this book are Open Access and distributed under the Creative Commons Attribution (CC BY) license. The book as a whole is distributed by MDPI under the terms and conditions of the Creative Commons Attribution-NonCommercial-NoDerivs (CC BY-NC-ND) license.

Contents

About the Editor vii

Junrui Zhou, Xuan Chen, Zhiming Wang and Qiuping Li
Couple-Based Communication Interventions for Cancer Patient–Spousal Caregiver Dyads' Psychosocial Adaptation to Cancer: A Systematic Review
Reprinted from: *Healthcare* 2023, 11, 236, doi:10.3390/healthcare11020236 1

Sanja D Tomić, Goran Malenković, Armin Šljivo, Ermina Mujičić and Slobodan Tomić
The Role of Resilience in the Relationship between Sociodemographic, Clinical Characteristics, and Social Support among Breast Cancer Patients in Serbia
Reprinted from: *Healthcare* 2023, 11, 3184, doi:10.3390/healthcare11243184 26

Su Jeong Yi, Ku Sang Kim, Seunghee Lee and Hyunjung Lee
Effects of Post Traumatic Growth on Successful Aging in Breast Cancer Survivors in South Korea: The Mediating Effect of Resilience and Intolerance of Uncertainty
Reprinted from: *Healthcare* 2023, 11, 2843, doi:10.3390/healthcare11212843 41

Inmaculada Valero-Cantero, Cristina Casals, Milagrosa Espinar-Toledo, Francisco Javier Barón-López, Nuria García-Agua Soler and María Ángeles Vázquez-Sánchez
Effects of Music on the Quality of Life of Family Caregivers of Terminal Cancer Patients: A Randomised Controlled Trial
Reprinted from: *Healthcare* 2023, 11, 1985, doi:10.3390/healthcare11141985 51

Mafalda Martins Cardoso, Cristina Lavareda Baixinho, Gilberto Tadeu Reis Silva and Óscar Ferreira
Nursing Interventions in the Perioperative Pathway of the Patient with Breast Cancer: A Scoping Review
Reprinted from: *Healthcare* 2023, 11, 1717, doi:10.3390/healthcare11121717 64

Raquel Veiga-Seijo and Cristina Gonzalez-Martin
Foot Health in People with Cancer Undergoing Chemotherapy: A Scoping Review
Reprinted from: *Healthcare* 2023, 11, 1588, doi:10.3390/healthcare11111588 75

Inmaculada Valero-Cantero, Cristina Casals, Milagrosa Espinar-Toledo, Francisco Javier Barón-López, Francisco Javier Martínez-Valero and María Ángeles Vázquez-Sánchez
Cancer Patients' Satisfaction with In-Home Palliative Care and Its Impact on Disease Symptoms
Reprinted from: *Healthcare* 2023, 11, 1272, doi:10.3390/healthcare11091272 92

Tzu-Ting Chang, Shu-Yuan Liang and John Rosenberg
Burden of Family Caregivers of Patients with Oral Cancer in Home Care in Taiwan
Reprinted from: *Healthcare* 2023, 11, 1107, doi:10.3390/healthcare11081107 104

Yoshiko Kitamura, Hisao Nakai, Yukie Maekawa, Hisako Yonezawa, Kazuko Kitamura and Tomoe Hashimoto et al.
Caregiver Burden among Family Caregivers of Cancer Survivors Aged 75 Years or Older in Japan: A Pilot Study
Reprinted from: *Healthcare* 2023, 11, 473, doi:10.3390/healthcare11040473 114

Hyun-Jung Lee, Bom-Mi Park, Mi-Jin Shin and Do-Yeon Kim
Therapeutic Communication Experiences of Nurses Caring for Patients with Hematology
Reprinted from: *Healthcare* 2022, 10, 2403, doi:10.3390/healthcare10122403 126

Yoshiko Kitamura, Hisao Nakai, Tomoe Hashimoto, Yuko Morikawa and Yoshiharu Motoo
Correlation between Quality of Life under Treatment and Current Life Satisfaction among Cancer Survivors Aged 75 Years and Older Receiving Outpatient Chemotherapy in Ishikawa Prefecture, Japan
Reprinted from: *Healthcare* **2022**, *10*, 1863, doi:10.3390/healthcare10101863 . . . . **141**

About the Editor

Qiuping Li

Professor Li Qiuping has been engaged in medical education and research for a long time. The main research directions are nursing education, digestive diseases, and cancer clinical research, and the research content is mainly concerned with the development and evaluation of supportive psychological intervention models for cancer patients and their family caregivers.

Systematic Review

Couple-Based Communication Interventions for Cancer Patient–Spousal Caregiver Dyads' Psychosocial Adaptation to Cancer: A Systematic Review

Junrui Zhou, Xuan Chen, Zhiming Wang and Qiuping Li *

Wuxi School of Medicine, Jiangnan University, Wuxi 214122, China
* Correspondence: 8166024040@jiangnan.edu.cn or liqp@163.com

Abstract: (1) Background: Effective communication among couples in which one has been diagnosed with cancer is critical to improve their psychosocial adaptation to cancer. The objective of this review was to explore the characteristics and measurement outcomes of existing couple-based communication interventions in the cancer context. (2) Methods: Eight electronic databases were searched from database initiation to August 2022 to identify eligible articles. Hand searching was also performed on the included articles' reference lists and authors. (3) Results: A total of 14 intervention studies were eligible to be included in this review. Cancer couples with distress or communication problems before intervention were more likely to benefit from the couple-based communication interventions. Positive outcomes were reported, including an improvement in relationship functioning (including mutual communication, intimacy, and relationship satisfaction) and individual functioning (including a decline of anxiety, depression and cancer-related concerns, and an increase in psychological adjustment and quality of life). (4) Conclusions: These findings supported the importance of improving mutual communication behaviors to promote cancer patient–spousal caregiver dyads' psychosocial adaptation to cancer. While most included studies were conducted in western countries and the sample size was relatively small, more research is warranted to develop more efficacious couple-based communication interventions.

Keywords: communication; intervention; program; cancer; couple; patient; spousal caregiver; adaptation

1. Introduction

According to updated global cancer statistics, approximately 19.3 million new cancer cases and an estimated 9.9 million cancer deaths occurred in 2020 for 36 types of cancers in 185 countries [1]. Furthermore, the global incidence of cancer is expected to increase to 28.4 million in 2040 [1]. According to an assessment by the World Health Organization (WHO), cancer was the first or second leading cause of death for the majority of countries in the world during the period from 2000 to 2019 [2]. The high incidence and mortality of cancer suggest that cancer-related issues are still a primary global disease burden. For those cancer patients who are married or in a committed relationship, patients and their spousal caregivers (SCs) generally experienced mutually related adaptation outcomes, such as self-efficacy, mental health, role adjustment, marital satisfaction, and quality of life (QOL) [3]. A study conducted by Lin et al., which focused on colorectal cancer patients (CPs) and their SCs, also found that CPs were positively related to their SCs, and vice versa [4]. Given the reciprocal influence among CPs and SCs, a growing number of researchers have advised to view cancer from a relational or dyadic perspective [5–7]. Kayser et al. [8] regard cancer as a "we-disease", which distinguished ownership of cancer. "We-disease" means that CPs and their SCs regard cancer as theirs and take efforts to communally cope with cancer-related stress as a couple [8]. Badr et al. [9] explored the effect of pronoun use during the natural communication context on a couple's psychosocial adaptation to head and neck cancer. They reported that more usage of first-person plural pronouns (e.g., we and ours) was related to a reduction in couples' distress, while more usage of first-person singular pronouns (e.g., I and mine) was related to couples' lower levels of marital satisfaction, which further supported the view that it is necessary and important to view CPs and SCs as CP–SC dyads.

Mutual communication plays a critical role in the psychosocial adaptation to cancer for CP–SC dyads. A review, which explored cancer couples' mutual impacts, reported that communication may be the fundamental element of the three concepts (which included "communication", "reciprocal influence", and "caregiver–patient congruence"), and better communication may facilitate an improvement in the other two concepts [3]. In addition, another review explored the impact paths of communication (among CPs and their family caregivers) on the adjustment to cancer based on 116 relevant studies [10]. Theoretical and empirical evidence supported the view that communication could impact the adjustment to cancer through at least three paths [10]. First, open communication could facilitate better coping through discussing and implementing methods of problem-solving, and further improve the adjustment to cancer. Second, as a kind of interactive coping mechanism (e.g., seeking support from spouses, discussing feelings and making new future plans with partners), communication could directly impact the adjustment to cancer. Third, cycling back and forth between communication patterns and coping strategies could jointly impact further adjustments to cancer. Except for impact paths, different communication patterns would have a different influence on CP–SC dyads' psychosocial adaptations to cancer. Based on previous theories and empiric studies, Manne et al. [11] proposed the Relationship Intimacy Model (RIM), which views cancer from a relational perspective and regards the marital relationship as a resource for dyadic couples coping with cancer. RIM is a dyadic-level theory which aims to promote CP–SP dyads' psychosocial adaptation to cancer through strengthening relationship-enhancing behaviors (including reciprocal self-disclosure, partner responsiveness, and relationship engagement) and decreasing relationship-compromising behaviors (including avoidance, criticism, and pressure-withdraw). Studies reported that mutual constructive communication between CPs and SCs was associated with greater relationship satisfaction (RS) and reduced psychological distress and depression, whereas mutual avoidance, critical communication and pressure-withdraw were related to lower RS, greater psychological distress and depression, and reduced well-being and psychological adjustment [3,12]. In addition, RIM also hypothesizes that relationship-enhancing and relationship-compromising behaviors could indirectly impact dyads' psychosocial adaptation to cancer by changing their intimacy [11]. Studies which focused on prostate CP–SC dyads reported that mutual constructive communication reduced psychological distress by promoting intimacy [13], while mutual avoidance, holding back and patient demand–partner withdrawal decreased RS and/or increased psychological distress by reducing intimacy [14]. Based on the aforementioned evidence, communication could impact CP–SC dyads' psychosocial adaptation to cancer in different ways. In this review, the psychosocial adaptation is categorized into two aspects, including relationship and individual functioning. Relationship functioning involves mutual communication, intimacy and RS, while individual functioning includes negative functioning (e.g., psychological distress and depression) and positive functioning (e.g., well-being and psychological adjustment).

With accumulating attention to relational perspective in the cancer context, a burgeoning number of couple-based interventions have emerged [15,16]. Most of these interventions comprised communication skill training components [17]. Couple-based communication plays an important role in helping couples understand cancer experiences, engage in social support, discuss role and responsibility changes and promote communal coping with cancer [17,18]. A meta-analysis reported that couple-based interventions for improving CP–SC dyads' adaptation to cancer had small but beneficial effects (Cohen's d = 0.25–0.31 for CPs, and Cohen's d = 0.21–0.24 for SCs) [19]. The most common reasons for these small effects were different or absent theoretical formats, varied intervention approaches and diverse measurements of outcomes [19]. Luo [20] provided multiple topics and comprehensive components for colorectal CP–SC dyads in her intervention study, and suggested that more focused content may make interventions more effective (e.g., focusing on couples' communication skills). At present, a systematic review assessing the effect of couple-based communication interventions on CP–SC dyads' psychosocial adaptation to cancer is lacking. In addition, a summary of the characteristics of the existing interventions is still needed to refine couple-based communication interventions for CP–SC dyads. Therefore, this review aims to (a) summarize the approach and contents of couple-based communication interventions in the cancer context, (b) explore these interventions' feasibility and acceptability, (c) review their impact on couples' relationship and/or individual functioning and (d) identify future research directions.

2. Methods

2.1. Search Methods for Eligible Articles

This review was performed in accordance with the PRISMA (Preferred Reporting Items for Systematic Reviews and Meta-Analyses) guidelines. A systematic search was performed to find all eligible studies which were published in English or Chinese. Six English databases (including CINAHL, Cochrane, Embase, Medline, PsyINFO, PubMed) and two databases (including CNKI and Wanfang Data) from China were searched from database initiation to August 2022. For the six English databases, the following key terms and their synonyms, which were limited to the title or abstract, were used: "cancer" or "tumor" or "oncology" AND "couple" or "spouse" or "partner" AND "communication" or "conservation" or "emotional disclosure" AND "program" or "training" or "education" or "intervention". Regarding the two Chinese databases, we used " 肿瘤" (tumor) or " 癌症" (cancer) AND " 夫妻" (couple) or " 配偶" (spouse) or " 伴侣" (partner) AND " 沟通" (communication) or " 交流" (conversation) AND " 干预" (intervention) or " 健康教育" (healthy education) as key words to search for eligible studies. For the purpose of finding as many relevant articles as possible, the outcome measures (e.g., "relationship satisfaction" or "psychological distress") were not included in the search terms, but they were considered during the selection process according to the inclusion and exclusion criteria. A manual search of reference lists of included studies and the relevant authors was also conducted to find additional eligible studies. Figure 1 shows a flowchart of the searching and selection process.

2.2. Selection Criteria for Identifying Articles

The inclusion criteria were as follows: (1) target population of studies was couples in which one had a diagnosis of any type of cancer; (2) interventions specially focused on couple-based communication components; (3) both the patients' and spouses' relationship and/or individual functioning were measured; (4) studies were completely published in peer-reviewed journals in English or Chinese.

The exclusion criteria were as follows: (1) except for SCs, informal caregivers also included other family members or friends; (2) interventions focused on CPs or SCs, but not CP–SC dyads; (3) interventions paid attention to other components (e.g., mindfulness training), instead of focusing on couple-based communication skill training; (4) studies were protocols, reviews, theses, conference proceedings or editorials.

2.3. Data Extraction and Synthesis

Two tables were used to fully extract and synthesize important information in the included studies. In Table 1, we primarily summarized the characteristics of the intervention articles, including the author, published year, country where the study was conducted, study aims, study design, characteristics of cancer and participants, theoretical framework, intervention component and dosage and delivery format. In Table 2, we synthesized the included studies' measurement tools and intervention outcomes.

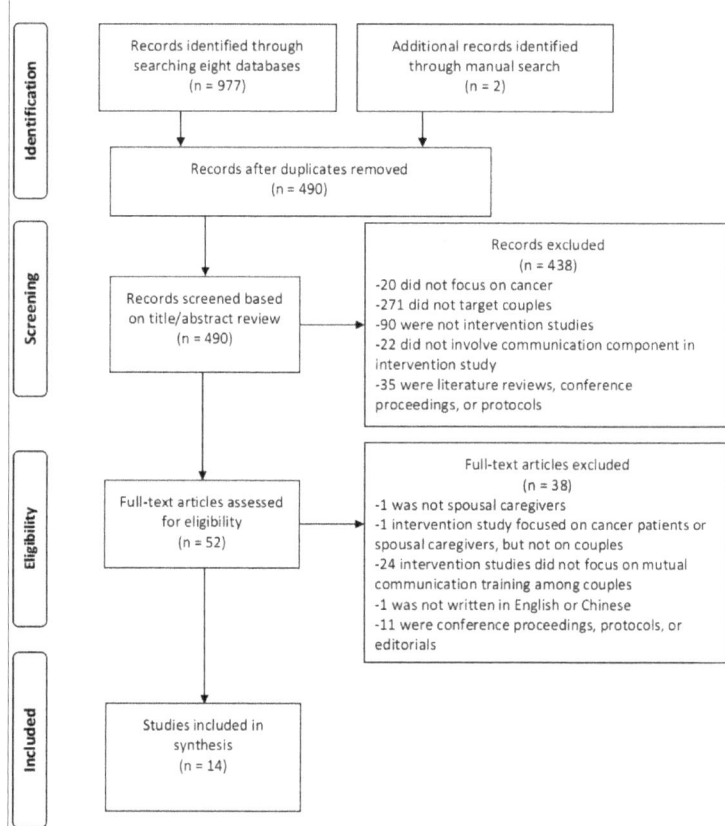

Figure 1. The flow diagram on identifying eligible articles in the literature.

2.4. Quality Assessment

We selected and used the Effective Public Health Practice Project (EPHPP) to assess the QR of included articles in this review. The EPHPP is a universal and comprehensive scale to examine bias in aspects of selection, design, confounders, data collection methods and withdrawals and dropouts for a series of study designs [21]. In addition, the EPHPP is regarded as a useful tool for systematic reviews that focus on intervention studies [22]. Table 3 provides detailed information of this assessment tool and the QR of included studies.

Notably, two trained reviewers independently extracted and synthesized data, and assessed the QR of the included studies. Discrepancies were resolved by the two reviewers through discussion until a consensus opinion was reached.

Table 1. Characteristics of included studies.

Author (Year) Country [Reference]	Study Aims	Study Design	Cancer Diagnosis (Stages); Characteristic and No. of Participants	Theoretical Framework	Intervention Content and Dosage	Delivery Format (Who and How)
Fergus et al. (2014) Canada [23]	-To assess feasibility and acceptability of the program; -To explore improved areas of participants after completing the program.	Single group study	Breast cancer (stages 0–3); All eligible participants regardless of level of relationship and individual functioning before intervention; Intervention Group (IG): 16 dyads.	-Developmental model of couple adaptation to illness (Rolland); -Theory of healthy relationship functioning (Gottman); -Models of dyadic coping (Bodenmann).	**Reciprocal self-disclosure:** (1) disclosure of own and partner's preference and experience through answering a series of topics (including cancer); (2) review and discuss own turning-toward and turning-away behaviors. **Partner responsiveness:** **Relationship engagement:** (1) communicate individual and relationship strengths; (2) think metaphorically about cancer and create a visual representation of cancer to fortify sense of "we-ness"; (3) watch video to learn sharing self-concerns and understand partner's perspective; (4) co-construct a relationship line about couple's pivotal events/periods and identify new life goals; (5) communally communicate with facilitators through the private website's 'Dialogue Room' discussion board; six modules (once weekly) within eight weeks.	-Mental health professional; -Online and telephone.
Fergus et al. (2022) Canada [24]	-To explore effect of the program on couple's relationship and individual functioning.	Randomized controlled trial (RCT)	Breast cancer (stages 0–3); All eligible participants, regardless of level of relationship and individual functioning before intervention; IG: 31 dyads; Control group (CG): 36 dyads.	-Systemic constructivist metatheory; -Developmental model of couple adaptation to illness (Rolland); -Theory of healthy relationship functioning (Gottman).	**Reciprocal self-disclosure:** (1) the same as the one (Fergus et al. [23]). **Partner responsiveness:** (1) the same as the one (Fergus et al. [23]). **Relationship engagement:** (1) discuss each physically pleasurable shared time and practice sensate focus exercise; (2) remaining contents were the same as the one (Fergus et al. [23]); six modules (once weekly) within eight weeks.	-Mental health professional; -Online and telephone.
Fergus et al. (2022) Canada [25]	-To assess acceptability of the couplelinks online program; -To explore gains of participants.	Single group study	Breast cancer (stages 0–3); All eligible participants regardless of relationship and individual functioning before intervention; IG: 30 dyads	-Systemic constructivist metatheory; -Developmental model of couple adaptation to illness (Rolland); -Theory of healthy relationship functioning (Gottman).	Intervention contents and dosage were the same as the one (Fergus et al. [24]).	-Mental health professional; -Online and telephone.

Table 1. Cont.

Author (Year) Country [Reference]	Study Aims	Study Design	Cancer Diagnosis (Stages); Characteristic and No. of Participants	Theoretical Framework	Intervention Content and Dosage	Delivery Format (Who and How)
Gremore et al. (2020) USA [26]	-To test feasibility and acceptability of a couple-based supportive communication (CSC) intervention; -To explore efficacy of CSC.	RCT	Head and neck cancer (stages 1–4a); All eligible participants regardless of relationship and individual functioning before intervention; -IG: 10 dyads; -CG: 10 dyads.	-Social-cognitive processing theory; -Relationship intimacy model (RIM).	**Reciprocal self-disclosure:** (1) express own vulnerable feelings. **Partner responsiveness:** (1) patiently listen to partner's disclosure and response with empathy and validation. **Relationship engagement:** (1) highlight individual and relationship strengths; (2) communicate supportively to understand problems rather than transitioning too quickly to problem-solving communication; (3) identify frequency of received and preferred support through completing support in intimate relationship rating scale (SIRRS); (4) review supportive communication skills and discuss transition to survivorship phase. **Relationship-compromising behaviors:** (1) block negative behaviors (e.g., invalidation); four sessions (each 75 min).	-Psychologist; -In person or video conference.
Manne et al. (2011) USA [27]	-To examine effects of the intimacy-enhancing therapy (IET) intervention; -To evaluate the role of baseline outcome variables in effects of IET on couples' relationship and psychological functioning.	RCT	Prostate cancer (stages 1–2); All eligible participants regardless of level of relationship and individual functioning before intervention; -IG: 37 dyads; -CG: 34 dyads.	-RIM.	**Reciprocal self-disclosure:** (1) improve couple's ability to comfortably share their cancer-related thoughts and feelings. **Partner responsiveness:** (1) improve mutual understanding. **Relationship engagement:** (1) improve constructive communication about cancer-related concerns, mutual support, and emotional intimacy; (2) complete in-session skill practice and home assignments; five sessions (each 90 min) within 8 weeks.	-Therapists; -In person.
Mowll et al. (2015) Australia [28]	-To explore feasibility and acceptability of patients dignity inventory couple interview (PDI-CI) intervention; -To determine effect of PDI-CI on couples.	Single group study	Cancer (advanced); All eligible participants regardless of level of relationship and individual functioning before intervention; IG: 9 dyads.	Not reported	**Reciprocal self-disclosure:** (1) individually complete PDI based on their own perception of patient's situation. **Relationship engagement:** (1) review results and identify concurrence and discordance with the psychologist, facilitate matched communication; one session (60 min).	-Psychologist; -In person.

Table 1. Cont.

Author (Year) Country [Reference]	Study Aims	Study Design	Cancer Diagnosis (Stages); Characteristic and No. of Participants	Theoretical Framework	Intervention Content and Dosage	Delivery Format (Who and How)
Porter et al. (2009) USA [29]	-To explore efficacy of partner-assisted emotional disclosure intervention comparing with providing cancer-related information.	RCT	Gastrointestinal (GI) cancer (stages 2–4); All eligible participants regardless of relationship and individual functioning before intervention; IG: 65 dyads; CG: 65 dyads.	Not reported	**Unidirectional self-disclosure:** (1) patients list their cancer-related concerns and disclose their own cancer-related events and feelings in as much detail as possible; **Unidirectional partner responsiveness:** (1) partners reflectively listen to patients' disclosure, try to understand cancer experience in patients' place, and avoid problem-solving, reassurance or advice giving; (2) identify helpful partner responses. **Relationship-compromising behaviors:** (1) identify unhelpful partner responses; four sessions (the first 75 min, the last three 45 min each) within four to eight weeks.	-Social worker or psychologist; -In person.
Porter et al. (2012) USA [30]	-To explore efficacy of partner-assisted emotional disclosure intervention comparing with providing cancer-related information; -To determine process variables that may influence the intervention effects.	RCT	GI cancer (stages 2–4); All eligible participants regardless of level of relationship and individual functioning before intervention; IG: 65 dyads; CG: 65 dyads.	Not reported	Intervention contents and dosage were the same as the one (Porter et al. [29]).	-Social workers or psychologists; -In person.
Porter et al. (2012) USA [31]	-To explore couples' experience in partner-assisted emotional disclosure intervention; -To determine variables associated with ratings of couples' communication.	Single group study	GI cancer (stages 2–4); All eligible participants regardless of level relationship and individual functioning before intervention; IG: 47 dyads.	Not reported	Intervention contents and dosage were the same as the one (Porter et al. [29]) above.	-Social workers or psychologists; -In person.
Shields et al. (2004) USA [32]	-To assess feasibility of the group intervention; -To explore efficacy of the group intervention.	Three groups study	Breast cancer (all stages); All eligible participants regardless of level of relationship and individual functioning before intervention; **2-session:** 12 dyads; **1-session:** 22 dyads; CG: 11 dyads.	Not reported	**Reciprocal self-disclosure:** (1) express cancer-related experience, cognition and emotions; (2) patients and partners express their own bridges and barriers to communicate with the other separately. **Partner responsiveness:** (1) listen supportively to partner's disclosure and gain new insights into their experience. **Relationship engagement:** (1) discuss bridges and barriers as a couple; (2) co-construct a relationship line about up or down times, plan for their life post-cancer and share and discuss the relationship line with other couples; 2-session group intervention: two sessions (each four hours); 1-session group intervention: one session (four hours) which was eliminated part of "bridges and barriers".	-Not reported; -Offline group intervention.

Table 1. Cont.

Author (Year) Country [Reference]	Study Aims	Study Design	Cancer Diagnosis (Stages); Characteristic and No. of Participants	Theoretical Framework	Intervention Content and Dosage	Delivery Format (Who and How)
Manne et al. (2019) USA [33]	-To compare the impact of IET, a general health and wellness (GHW) intervention, and Usual Care (UC) on couples' relationship and psychological functioning.	RCT	Prostate cancer (stages 1–3); Ones who had distress before intervention; IG: 80 dyads CG: GHW: 76 dyads; UC: 81 dyads.	-RIM.	**Reciprocal self-disclosure:** (1) disclosure of cancer experience and sources of distress and create a list of cancer concerns; (2) express support needs. **Partner responsiveness:** (1) respond with empathy and validation. **Relationship engagement:** (1) learn problem-solving model; (2) practice speaking, listening and problem-solving skill with a cancer concern during in-session exercise and home assignment, and practice sensate focus exercise at home; (3) review skills and challenges, and troubleshoot future issues; six sessions (each 90 min) and one booster call (30–45 min).	-Psychologist or social worker; -In person and telephone.
Porter et al. (2017) USA [34]	-To determine the feasibility and acceptability of the couples communication skills training (CCST) intervention; -To explore effects of CCST compared with an educational intervention (HLI).	RCT	GI cancer (stage 4); Ones who presented holding back pattern before intervention; IG: 15 dyads; CG: 17 dyads.	Not reported	**Reciprocal self-disclosure:** (1) share thoughts and feelings about a series of cancer-related topics. **Partner responsiveness:** (1) accept and affirm partners' feelings and perspectives. **Relationship engagement:** (1) try to make a cancer-related decision through communication skills; (2) review progress during treatment and identify future issues related to communicating about cancer; six sessions (each 60 min).	-Social workers; -Video conference.
Porter et al. (2018) USA [35]	-To determine themes discussed by couples during CCST intervention.	Single group study	GI cancer (advanced); Ones who presented holding back pattern before intervention; IG: 12 dyads.	Not reported	Intervention contents and dosage were the same as the one (Porter et al. [34]).	-Social workers; -Video conference.

Table 1. Cont.

Author (Year) Country [Reference]	Study Aims	Study Design	Cancer Diagnosis (Stages); Characteristic and No. of Participants	Theoretical Framework	Intervention Content and Dosage	Delivery Format (Who and How)
Su et al. (2022) China [36]	-To explore feasibility and efficacy of CCST.	RCT	Gastric cancer (stages 3–4); Couples who presented cancer-related communication problem before intervention; IG: 44 dyads; CG: 43 dyads.	Not reported	**Reciprocal self-disclosure:** (1) express experience, thoughts and feelings sincerely through a cancer-related topic. **Partner responsiveness:** (1) reflectively listen to partner's emotional disclosure, accept partner's feelings and avoid giving advice quickly. **Relationship engagement:** (1) practice communication skills in each session; (2) try to make a cancer-related decision through communication skills; (3) write and read the letter of thanks for each other, review progress and discuss coping strategies for future cancer-related communication problems. **Relationship-compromising behaviors:** (1) point out couples' unreasonable communication behaviors; five sessions (each 60 min) within five to seven weeks.	-Psychologist and nursing postgraduate; -In person.

Table 2. Outcomes of included studies. Symbols # and * could help us to distinguish whether the tools examine patients or spousal caregivers clearly.

Author (Year) Country [Reference]	Outcome Measurements (Measurement Intervals)	Program Evaluation Outcomes (Feasibility, Acceptability)	Intervention Effects ($p < 0.05$ Indicates Statistical Significance)	
			Relationship Functioning	Individual Functioning
Fergus et al. (2014) Canada [23]	**Feasibility** -Recruitment and completion rate. **Acceptability** -Treatment Satisfaction Questionnaire (TSQ); At post-treatment. **Primary outcome measures** -Interview; At post-treatment.	**Feasibility** -Recruitment rate: 57.14%; completion rate: 62.5% of participants completed all modules; **Acceptability** -85% of couples satisfied with the program; the majority of couples regarded facilitator as helpful and effective; 61% of couples agreed that the website was easy to use; 55% of couples regarded the program as convenient; -Limitations: program disrupted couple's usual routine, lacked profoundness and was impersonal.	**Within-group comparison of pre–post change** -The program opened couple's communication channel, enhanced couple's communication skill and improved meaningful cancer-related discussion; -Couples learned more relationship knowledge, perceived higher closeness with each other, and affirmed relationship strengths.	

Table 2. Cont.

Author (Year) Country [Reference]	Outcome Measurements (Measurement Intervals)	Program Evaluation Outcomes (Feasibility, Acceptability)	Intervention Effects ($p < 0.05$ Indicates Statistical Significance)	
			Relationship Functioning	Individual Functioning
Fergus et al. (2022) Canada [24]	**Feasibility** -Recruitment, retention and completion rate. **Primary outcome measures Relationship functioning:** *positive dyadic coping:* Positive Dyadic Coping 19-item subscale of the Dyadic Coping Inventory; *relationship satisfaction (RS):* Revised-Dyadic Adjustment Scale (DAS), Kansas Marital Satisfaction Survey; *self-perceived own dyadic coping;* The Breast Cancer and Relationship Measure; **Individual functioning:** *anxiety and depression:* Hospital Anxiety and Depression Scale (HADS); At baseline, post-treatment and 3-month follow-up.	**Feasibility** -Recruitment rate: 89.3%; retention rate: 89% at post-treatment, 77% at 3-month follow-up; completion rate: all couples in IG completed at least five sessions.	**Within-group comparison of pre–post change** -Couples reported positive change in positive dyadic coping ($b = 2.40$, $p = 0.032$, Cohen's $d = 0.24$) and perceived own dyadic coping ($b = 3.93$, $p = 0.04$, Cohen's $d = 0.23$) in IG from baseline to post-treatment, but not from baseline to 3-month follow-up; -There was no significant change in couples' RS regardless of treatment arms or follow-up periods.	**Within-group comparison of pre–post change** -Couples reported less anxiety from baseline to 3-month follow-up ($p = 0.03$), but not from baseline to post-treatment in IG, while couples had reduced anxiety from baseline to post-treatment ($b = -0.58$, $p = 0.046$) and from baseline to 3-month follow-up ($b = -0.67$, $p = 0.022$) in CG; -There was no positive change in depression regardless of treatment arms or follow-up periods.
Fergus et al. (2022) Canada [25]	**Acceptability** -TSQ; open-ended questions to ask most and least helpful parts of the program, and feedback on the psychoeducational articles and videos. **Primary outcome measures** -Interview; After 1–2 weeks after post-treatment.	**Acceptability** -Couples satisfied with the program, while females reported higher satisfaction than males (Cohen's $d = 0.42$, $p = 0.01$); -The favorable parts were varied (e.g., "the variety of activity", "the role playing" or "facing cancer as a unified front"), while limitations were lacking in-person contact, and novel learning.	**Within-group comparison of pre–post change** -Couples started to communicate with each other again, learned communication skills, spent quality time together, obtained insight into their relationship and perceived that they were "in this together".	
Gremore et al. (2020) USA [26]	**Feasibility** -Recruitment, retention and completion rates. **Acceptability** -Client Satisfaction Questionnaire (CSQ); -Questions to assess most and least helpful aspects at post-treatment. **Primary outcome measures Relationship functioning:** RS: DAS; *intimacy:* Miller Social Intimacy Scale (MSIS); **Individual functioning:** *post-traumatic stress:* Impact of Events Scale (IES) – Revised; *anxiety:* Emotional Distress Scale–Anxiety; *depression:* The Center for Epidemiological Studies-Depression (CES-D); *patient quality of life (QOL):* Functional Assessment of Cancer Therapy–Head and Neck #; *caregiver QOL:* Caregiver Quality of Life Index–Cancer *; Baseline, at post-treatment and 6-month follow-up.	**Feasibility** -Recruitment rate: 33.3%, retention rate: 80% for IG, 90% for CG; completion rate: 80% of IG participants and 90% of CG participants completed all sessions, 90% of participants in both IG and CG completed post-treatment, and 90% of IG participants and 80% of CG participants completed 6-month follow-up measures. **Acceptability** -CPs and their SCs were satisfied with the intervention, communicating about their feelings was helpful, but questionnaire measures were too long.	**Between-group comparisons of pre–post change** -CPs reported no more improvement in RS regardless of follow-up period, but more improvement in intimacy (Cohen's $d = 0.42$) at post-treatment in IG than CG but no difference at 6-month follow-up; -SCs had more improvement in RS (Cohen's $d = 0.53$ and 0.47) and intimacy (Cohen's $d = 0.45$ and 0.24) at post-treatment and 6-month follow-up respectively to IG than CG.	**Between-group comparisons of pre- and post-change** -CPs had more anxiety ($t = 2.78$, $p < 0.05$) and depression ($t = 2.40$, $p < 0.05$) at baseline in IG than CG. -CPs reported more improvement in post-traumatic stress (Cohen's $d = 0.22$) and QOL (Cohen's $d = 0.48$) at 6-month follow-up but not at post-treatment, and more improvement in anxiety (Cohen's $d = 0.65$ and 1.17) and depression (Cohen's $d = 0.33$ and 0.91) at post-treatment and 6-month follow-up, respectively, in IG than CG; -SCs had more improvement in post-traumatic stress (Cohen's $d = 0.88$ and 0.87), anxiety (Cohen's $d = 0.57$ and 0.47), depression (Cohen's $d = 0.45$ and 0.61) and QOL (Cohen's $d = 0.22$ and 0.31) at post-treatment and 6-month follow-up, respectively, in IG than CG.

Table 2. Cont.

Author (Year) Country [Reference]	Outcome Measurements (Measurement Intervals)	Program Evaluation Outcomes (Feasibility, Acceptability)	Intervention Effects ($p < 0.05$ Indicates Statistical Significance)	
			Relationship Functioning	Individual Functioning
Manne et al. (2011) USA [27]	**Feasibility** -Recruitment, retention and completion rates. **Acceptability** -Questions for success of the intervention. **Primary outcome measures/Moderators** -Relationship functioning: *self-disclosure*: 3-item measure; *perceived partner disclosure*: 3-item measure; *perceived partner responsiveness*: 4-item measure; *mutual constructive communication*: The Constructive Communication subscale of the Communications Pattern Questionnaire (CPQ); *demand-withdraw communication*: The Demand-Withdraw subscale of the CPQ; *intimacy*: The Personal Assessment of Intimacy in Relationships; *RS*: DAS; -Individual functioning: *psychological distress*: The Psychological Distress scale of the Mental Health Inventory (MHI); *psychological well-being*: The Psychological Well-Being scale of MHI; *cancer-specific distress*: IES; *cancer concerns*: 10 self-report questions; Baseline, at eight weeks post-baseline.	**Feasibility** -Recruitment rate: 20.8%; retention rate: 94.6% for IG, 80.9% for CG; completion rate: 70.3% of participants completed all sessions. **Acceptability** -CPs and their SCs reported that sessions were quite successful.	**Between-group comparisons of pre- and post-change** -CPs reported higher scores of self-disclosure ($t = 3.50$, $p < 0.001$), perceived partner disclosure ($t = 3.27$, $p = 0.002$), and perceived partner responsiveness ($t = 3.26$, $p = 0.034$) in IG than CG when these variables were low before intervention; lower scores of self-disclosure ($t = -2.34$, $p = 0.022$) in IG than CG when the variable was high before intervention; -SCs had higher scores of mutual constructive communication ($t = 3.70$, $p < 0.001$), intimacy ($t = 3.42$, $p = 0.001$) and RS ($t = 3.94$, $p < 0.001$) in IG than CG when these variables were low before intervention; lower scores of demand-withdraw communication ($t = -2.34$, $p = 0.023$), intimacy ($t = -2.49$, $p = 0.015$) and RS ($t = -2.12$, $p = 0.038$) in IG than CG when these variables were high before intervention.	**Between-group comparisons of pre-post change** -CPs reported fewer cancer-related concerns ($t = -2.34$, $p = 0.022$) in IG than CG when the variable was high at baseline; -SCs had less cancer-specific distress ($t = -2.31$, $p = 0.024$) in IG than CG when the variable was high at baseline.
Manne et al. (2019) USA [33]	**Feasibility** -Recruitment, retention and completion rates. **Acceptability** -14 items assessed helpfulness and importance of the intervention. At three months post-baseline. **Primary outcome measures** -Relationship functioning: *RS*: DAS; -Individual functioning: *general psychological adjustment*: MHI-38; *depression*: The Patient Health Questionnaire-9 (PHQ-9); *cancer-specific distress*: IES; *cancer-related concerns*: 10 self-report questions. Baseline, at five weeks post-baseline, at three months post-baseline, and at six months post-baseline.	**Feasibility** -Recruitment rate: 15.2%; retention rate: 90% for IG, 78.9% for general health and wellness intervention, 85.2% for Usual Care group; complete rate: 86% of IG couples and 73.6% of CG couples attended five or six sessions; 89–92% CPs and 89–91% SCs completed homework; **Acceptability** -Satisfaction ratings were high for couples in both IG and CG.	**Within-group comparison of pre- and post-change** -CPs had no significant change in RS in three treatment arms over time; -SCs perceived improvement in RS in IG from baseline to five weeks post-baseline (Cohen's $d = 0.22$), but not at other follow-up periods.	**Within-group comparison of pre- and post-change** -CPs and SCs had significant improvement in general psychological adjustment, depression, cancer-specific distress, cancer concerns at varied follow-up periods regardless of treatment arms.
Mowll et al. (2015) Australia [28]	**Feasibility** -Recruitment and retention rates; **Acceptability** -Interviews; At two weeks post-treatment; **Primary outcome measures** -Interviews; At two weeks post-treatment.	**Feasibility** -Recruitment rate: 35.3%; retention rate: 75%; **Acceptability** -Most participants like the intervention and obtained some benefits, while one patient thought that psychologist did not discuss enough for discordance.	**Within-group comparison of pre- and post-change** -Male CPs and male SCs had more opportunities to talk; -The intervention promoted validated communication among couples which promoted closeness, mutual understanding and support.	

11

Table 2. Cont.

Author (Year) Country [Reference]	Outcome Measurements (Measurement Intervals)	Program Evaluation Outcomes (Feasibility, Acceptability)	Intervention Effects ($p < 0.05$ Indicates Statistical Significance)	
			Relationship Functioning	Individual Functioning
Porter et al. (2009) USA [29]	**Feasibility** -Recruitment and retention rates; **Primary outcome measures** -Relationship functioning: *intimacy*: MSIS; *relationship quality*: Quality of Marriage Index (QMI); -Individual functioning: *psychological distress*: Profile of Mood States-Short Form (POMS-SF); Baseline, at post-treatment; **Moderator** -*holding back*: 10 self-report items #; Baseline.	**Feasibility** -Recruitment rate: 24.9%; retention rate: 86.7%; completion rate: 83.1% of participants completed post-treatment assessment.	**Between-group comparisons of pre- and post-change** -CPs and SCs reported more improvement in intimacy and relationship quality in IG than CG only when CPs had high holding back from discussing cancer-related concerns before intervention.	**Between-group comparisons of pre- and post-change** -CPs and SCs reported no significant change in psychological distress between treatment arms.
Porter et al. (2012) USA [30]	**Primary outcome measures** -Relationship functioning: *intimacy*: MSIS, *relationship quality*: QMI; -Individual functioning: *psychological distress*: POMS-SF; *holding back*: 10 self-reported items #; **Process variables** -*Negative affect*: Negative Affect Subscale #; *observational ratings of patient expressiveness during the treatment sessions*: Self-Feeling Awareness Scale (SFAS) #; Baseline, at post-treatment and 8-week follow-up.	Not reported	**Between-group comparisons of pre- and post-change** -CPs and SCs reported more increase in intimacy and relationship quality at post-treatment and eight weeks follow-up in IG than CG when CPs had high holding back before intervention; -High level of CPs' expression during sessions were related to promotion of couples' intimacy and relationship quality at post-treatment.	**Between-group comparisons of pre- and post-change** -CPs and SCs reported no significant change in individual functioning between treatment arms; -High level of CPs' negative affect immediately after each session were related to decline of couples' psychological distress at post-treatment.
Porter et al. (2012) USA [31]	**Primary outcome measures** -Relationship function: *communication*: SFAS #, the Acceptance of Other Scale *, Post-session Self-Report Measures of Communication; At each post-session. **Moderators** *relationship quality*: QMI; *intimacy*: MSIS; *perceived partner avoidance and criticism*: 13-item scale; *disclosure and holding back*: ten domains of concern regarding gastrointestinal cancer; *psychological distress*: POMS-SF; Baseline.	Not reported	**Within-group comparison of pre–post change** -CPs rarely directly talked about their emotion; -SCs generally provided instrumental support rather than responding to the CPs' emotion; -SCs were more possible to respond empathically when CPs were more expressive; -Empathic SCs were less likely to criticize their CPs; -CPs were rated as more expressive in IG when they reported lower relationship quality, higher partner avoidance, and higher holding back before intervention.	

Table 2. Cont.

Author (Year) Country [Reference]	Outcome Measurements (Measurement Intervals)	Program Evaluation Outcomes (Feasibility, Acceptability)	Intervention Effects ($p < 0.05$ Indicates Statistical Significance)	
			Relationship Functioning	Individual Functioning
Porter et al. (2017) USA [34]	**Feasibility** -Recruitment, retention and completion rates. **Acceptability** -CSQ; -Questions to assess the convenience of videoconference format, preference delivery format, and most and least helpful aspects of the intervention; At post-treatment. **Primary outcome measures** -Relationship functioning: *communication*: Problem Solving Communication subscale, Affective Communication subscale; *intimacy*: MSIS; RS: Revised-DAS; -Individual functioning: *cancer-related distress*: eight-item version of IES; *psychological growth*: Post-traumatic Growth Inventory (PTGI); *self-efficacy*: a standard self-efficacy scale; Baseline, at post-treatment.	**Feasibility** -Recruitment rate: 28%; retention rate: 80% for IG, 100% for CG; completion rate: 88% of participants completed all six sessions. **Acceptability** -Satisfaction ratings were high for CP and their SC in both treatment arms; -Participants reported highly satisfactory regarding videoconference format; rates of preference for formats of video conference, in person and telephone were 77%, 20% and 3%, respectively; most helpful aspect was listening skill.	**Between-group comparisons of pre–post change** -CPs reported more improvement in affective communication (*Cohen's d* = −0.35), problem-solving communication (*Cohen's d* = −0.50), intimacy (*Cohen's d* = 0.63), and RS (*Cohen's d* = 0.30) in IG than CG; -SCs perceived more improvement in RS (*Cohen's d* = 0.34) in IG than CG, but not for communication and intimacy.	**Between-group comparisons of pre–post change** -CPs reported more improvement on the PTGI Personal Strength subscale (*Cohen's d* = 0.36) in IG than CG, and greater increase in self-efficacy (*Cohen's d* = −0.22) and PTGI New Possibilities (*Cohen's d* = −0.37) in CG than IG; -SCs perceived more improvement on the PTGI relating to others (*Cohen's d* = 0.49) in IG than CG, and more increase in self-efficacy (*Cohen's d* = −0.25) in CG than IG; -No significant effect on cancer-related distress for CPs and SCs in IG than CG.
Porter et al. (2018) USA [35]	**Primary outcome measures** -Interviews; During the intervention.	Not reported	**Within-group comparison of pre- and post-change** -CPs and SCs discussed to attempt to maintain normal relationship with each other rather than being in the role of "patient" and "caregiver"; -CPs and SCs shared mutual understanding and addressed conflicts; -CPs desired to provide support to their SCs; -CPs and SCs discussed symptom-related emotional and practical considerations and made likely future treatment decisions; -CPs and SCs discussed death-related topics; -Couples highlighted importance of couple relationship for each other.	
Shields et al. (2004) USA [32]	**Feasibility** -Recruitment and completion rates. **Primary outcome measures** -Relationship functioning: RS: Revised-DAS; -Individual functioning: *mental health*: Mental Health Summary Score of The Medical Outcomes Study Short-Form (12 item scale) (SF-12); *cancer-related stress*: IES. Baseline, at post-treatment and 3-month follow-up.	**Feasibility** -Recruitment rate: 50%; completion rate: 82% of 2-session group, 73% of 1-session group, and 80% of comparison group completed time 3 assessment.	**Within-group comparisons of pre- and post-change** -CPs and SCs reported no visible change in RS in three study arms regardless of follow-up period.	**Within and between-group comparisons of pre- and post-change** -CPs had visible improvement of mental health and avoidance in 2-session group, but SCs had no visible change in each individual functioning in three study arms.

Table 2. Cont.

Author (Year) Country [Reference]	Outcome Measurements (Measurement Intervals)	Program Evaluation Outcomes (Feasibility, Acceptability)	Intervention Effects ($p < 0.05$ Indicates Statistical Significance)	
			Relationship Functioning	Individual Functioning
Su et al. (2022) China [36]	**Feasibility** -Recruitment and completion rates. **Primary outcome measures** -Relationship functioning; *communication*: Cancer-Related Communication Problem Scale (CRCP); *RS*: Relationship Assessment Scale (RAS); Baseline, at post-treatment.	**Feasibility** -Recruitment rate: 95.7% for IG, 93.5% for CG; completion rate: 90.9% of participants completed four to five sessions and 93.2% of participants completed home assignment.	**Within-group comparisons of pre- and post-change)** -CPs and SCs reported improvement in communication and RS in IG, but not in CG. **Between-group comparisons of pre- and post-change** -CPs and their SCs had more improvement in communication and RS at post-treatment in IG than CG.	

Table 3. Quality assessment of the included studies (n = 14).

Author; (Year); Country [Reference Number]	Selection Bias	Design	Confounders	Blinding	Data Collection	Dropouts	Quality Rating
Fergus et al. (2014) Canada [23]	W	M	W	W	W	M	W
Fergus et al. (2022) Canada [24]	S	S	S	M	M	S	S
Fergus et al. (2022) Canada [25]	S	M	M	M	W	S	M
Gremore et al. (2020) USA [26]	W	S	M	S	M	S	M
Manne et al. (2011) USA [27]	W	S	S	M	S	S	M
Manne et al. (2019) USA [33]	W	S	S	M	S	S	M
Mowll et al. (2015) Australia [28]	W	M	W	W	W	S	W
Porter et al. (2009) USA [29]	W	S	S	S	M	S	M
Porter et al. (2012) USA [30]	W	S	S	M	M	M	M

Table 3. *Cont.*

Author; (Year); Country [Reference Number]	Selection Bias	Design	Confounders	Blinding	Data Collection	Dropouts	Quality Rating
Porter et al. (2012) USA [31]	M	M	S	S	M	S	S
Porter et al. (2017) USA [34]	W	S	M	S	M	S	M
Porter et al. (2018) USA [35]	M	M	W	M	W	S	W
Shields et al. (2004) USA [32]	W	M	W	W	M	M	W
Su et al. (2022) China [36]	S	S	S	M	M	S	S

Selection bias: Strong—very likely to be representative of the target population and greater than 80% participation rate; Moderate—somewhat likely to be representative of the target population and 60–79% participation rate; Weak—all other responses or not stated. Design: Strong—RCT and CCT; Moderate—cohort analytic, case-control, cohort or an interrupted time series; Weak—all other designs or design not stated. Confounders: Strong—controlled for at least 80% of confounders; Moderate—controlled for 60–79% of confounders; Weak—confounders not controlled for, or not stated. Blinding: Strong—blinding of outcome assessor and study participants to intervention status and/or research question; Moderate—blinding of either outcome assessor or study participants; Weak—outcome assessor and study participants were aware of intervention status and/or research question. Data collection methods: Strong—tools were valid and reliable; Moderate—tools were valid but reliability not described; Weak—no evidence of validity or reliability. Withdrawals and dropouts: Strong—follow-up rate of >80% of participants; Moderate—follow-up rate of 60–79% of participants; Weak—follow-up rate of <60% of participants or withdrawals and dropouts not described. Quality rating: S: strong; M: moderate; W: weak. Strong: If a study had no weak ratings and at least four strong ratings, then it was considered strong; Moderate: If the study had fewer than four strong ratings and one weak rating, it was rated moderate; Weak: If a study had two or more weak ratings, it was considered weak.

3. Results

3.1. Process of Study Selection

A total of 979 articles were found in eight databases and after additional manual searching, and 489 duplicates were excluded using EndNote 20. The titles and abstracts of the remaining 490 articles were reviewed based on inclusion and exclusion criteria. Of the 490 studies, 438 studies were excluded and 52 articles remained to be reviewed for the full-text component. Finally, 14 studies were included in this review for analysis. Figure 1 shows detailed information on the selection process. The most common reasons why studies were removed were that target population of studies were not couples, articles were not intervention studies or interventions did not focus on couple-based communication components.

3.2. Result of Quality Assessment

Table 3 illustrates the quality assessment of the involved articles. Three, seven, and four articles were rated as "strong", "moderate" and "weak", respectively. The rating of "weak" was mainly owing to a low recruitment rate of the target population, not using a blinding strategy and controlling confounders, and using tools without evidence of validity or reliability. Although the QR of the studies was varied, we included all of them because they basically completed their study aims and met the selection criteria of this review.

3.3. Characteristics of Intervention

Most intervention studies included in this review were carried out in western countries, including the USA (n = 9, 64.3%), Canada (n = 3, 21.4%) and Australia (n = 1, 7.1%), while one was from China (7.1%). The designs of the intervention studies were randomized controlled trial (RCT) (n = 8, 57.1%), single-group study (n = 5, 35.7%) and three-group study (n = 1, 7.1%). The single-group study included a pre–post single-arm study and interviews for participants from the treatment arm only.

3.4. Characteristics of Participants

Of the 14 articles involved in this review, 13 focused on a single type of cancer with varied stages, including gastrointestinal cancer (n = 5, 41.7%), breast cancer (n = 4, 28.6%), prostate cancer (n = 2, 14.3%), head and neck cancer (n = 1, 7.1%) and gastric cancer (n = 1, 7.1%), while one targeted any type of cancer with an advanced stage (n = 1, 7.1%). Notably, of the 13 articles testing a single type of cancer, seven focused on non-gender-specific cancer, while six targeted gender-specific cancer (e.g., breast or prostate cancer). The articles' sample sizes differed, ranging from nine dyads to 237 dyads. Across the target population, 10 studies focused on participants regardless of the level of their relationship or individual functioning before the intervention [23–32], while four studies recruited those who had distress or cancer-related communication problems before the intervention [33–36]. In addition, ethnicity and education level of the majority of the participants in the included studies were Caucasian and college or higher, respectively.

3.5. Theoretical Framework of the Interventions

Six kinds of theoretical framework were used to instruct the research included in this review, including the developmental model of couple adaptation to illness [23–25], the theory of health relationship functioning [23–25], models of dyadic coping [23], systemic-constructive metatheory [24,25], social-cognitive processing theory [26] and RIM [26,27,33]. Among these theoretical frameworks, RIM was the most frequently demonstrated and was used to guide two kinds of intervention programs. Most included studies did not use a specific theoretical framework to guide their intervention, or some of those using a theoretical framework did not demonstrate how the framework guided their intervention in detail.

3.6. Intervention Content

In this review, interventions' contents were summarized according to RIM, including four aspects: reciprocal self-disclosure, partner responsiveness, relationship engagement and relationship-compromising behaviors [11]. All 14 studies included self-disclosure contents, which primarily aimed to guide couples to disclose cancer-related experiences, thoughts and feelings. Of the 14 studies, 11 studies trained reciprocal self-disclosure [23–28,32–36], while the remaining three studies trained CPs' unidirectional self-disclosure to their SCs [29–31]. Partner responsiveness contents were included in 13 studies [23–27,29–36], which mainly aimed to teach partners to become attentive listeners to help the other couple member feel understood and cared for. The main components included recording and discussing their own turning-toward and turning-away behaviors, patiently listening to their partner's emotional disclosure, accepting and affirming their thoughts and feelings, responding with empathy and validation and avoiding giving advice quickly. Three studies only focused on the SCs' unidirectional responsiveness to CPs [29–31]. Relationship engagement was defined as viewing cancer as a relational event and engaging in behaviors to maintain or strengthen the relationship in the context of cancer [11]. In this review, 11 studies included relationship engagement [23–28,32–36], comprising of practicing speaking and listening skills with cancer-related topics, improving problem-solving, highlighting individual and relationship strengths, enhancing a sense of "we-ness" in relation to cancer, co-constructing the relationship line about couples' pivotal events/periods, writing and reading thanks letter to each other and identifying new goals for the future. With regard to relationship-compromising behaviors, pointing out or blocking unreasonable communication behaviors was reported [26,29–31,36].

3.7. Delivery Format and Intervention Dosage

3.7.1. Delivery Format

The characteristics of the intervention deliverers were reported by 13 articles. Five articles' intervention deliverers were psychologists [23–26,28], four were psychologists or social workers [29–31,33], two were social workers [34,35], one was therapists [27], and one was psychologists and nurses [36]. The delivery formats of the 14 studies varied, including in-person (n = 6, 42.9%) [27–31,36], online and telephone (n = 3, 21.4%) [23–25], video conference (n = 2, 14.3%) [34,35], in-person and telephone (n = 1, 7.1%) [33], in-person or video conference (n = 1, 7.1%) [26] and offline group interventions (n = 1, 7.1%) [32].

3.7.2. Intervention Dosage

The number of modules/sessions in the 14 intervention studies was varied, ranging from one to six, with an average of 3.5. Of the 14 articles included in this review, 10 articles illustrated that each session generally lasted 60 to 90 min [26,27,29–36]. The length of each online module of three articles was chosen by the participants [23–25]. One study spent four hours in each session [28]. In addition, for the duration of the intervention, eight studies reported that the duration generally ranged from four to eight weeks, and the average value was six weeks [23–25,27,29–31,36]. Five articles did not mention the duration [26,32–35], while one study had only one session constructed during the first counselling session [28]. With regard to the follow-up periods, four studies had single follow-up timepoints, including eight weeks [30], three months [24,32] and six months after intervention [26], while another adopted multiple follow-up periods [33].

3.8. Feasibility and Acceptability

3.8.1. Feasibility

The feasibility of the interventions was assessed in 10 studies. Eight studies reported generally low recruitment rates that were less than 60% [23,26–29,32–34], while two studies had relatively high recruitment rates above 60% (including one online intervention program conducted in Canada [24] and one in-person intervention conducted in China [36]). The reasons why participants refused to take part in the intervention mainly involved them being too busy, too far away, too sick, lacking interest or lacking need. It is worth noting that studies showed relatively high retention rates (ranging from 75% to 100%), and relatively high completion rates, which were demonstrated by the fact that 62.5–100% of participants completed most modules/sessions, 89–93.2% of participants completed relevant practice and 73–90% of participants completed outcome measurements.

3.8.2. Acceptability

Seven studies examined the acceptability of their interventions. CPs and their SCs were highly satisfied with interventions [23,25,26,28,33,34] or viewed the intervention as quite successful [27]. Particularly, for one online intervention program, females reported higher satisfaction than males (Cohen's d = 0.42, p = 0.01) [25]. The favorable aspects of programs for participants encompassed communicating their own feelings [26], listening skill [34] and "the variety of activity", "the role playing" or "facing cancer as a unified front" [24]. In addition, limitations were also pointed out, including that the online intervention program lacked in-person contact [23,25], the questionnaire was too long [26] and the intervention lacked profoundness [23,28]. Approximately 60% of participants in the online intervention programs regarded website usage as convenient [23,25]. Another study reported that the rates of participants' preferences for delivery formats were 77%, 20%, and 3% for video conference, in-person and telephone interventions, respectively [34].

3.9. Intervention Outcomes

All 14 studies measured relationship functioning, such as mutual communication, intimacy, and RS, and/or individual functioning, including anxiety, depression, psychological distress, cancer concerns, psychological adjustment and QOL for CPs and their SCs. The detailed information of intervention outcomes can be found in Table 2. In this review, the outcomes of relationship and individual functioning were separately analyzed according to within- and between-group comparisons of pre–post change.

3.9.1. Effects on Relationship Functioning for Within-Group Comparisons of Pre–Post Change

Eight studies reported that CPs and/or their SCs experienced a significant improvement in their mutual communication [23–25,28,31,35,36], intimacy [23,25,28] and RS [23,25,33,35,36] in the intervention group (IG). For these significant outcomes, it was found that the interventions had a short-term (up to five weeks) impact on relationship functioning [33]. In addition, three studies reported that CPs and/or their SCs with distress or communication problems (e.g., holding back) before the intervention seemed to be more able to benefit from the interventions [33,35,36]. On the contrary, one online intervention [24] and another offline group intervention [32], which viewed RS as the primary outcome, did not improve the RS of either CPs or their SCs during multiple follow-up periods.

3.9.2. Effects on Relationship Functioning for Between-Group Comparisons of Pre–Post Change

Gremore et al. [26] reported that CPs and their SCs, regardless of their level of relationship and individual functioning before the intervention, experienced more improvement in intimacy and RS in the IG than the control group (CG), even at six months follow-up. Another five studies showed that the intervention positively impacted relationship functioning only when CPs and/or their SCs had a low or negative functioning before the intervention [27,29,30,34,36]. Of the five studies, one demonstrated that CPs reported higher scores of self-disclosure (t = 3.50, p < 0.001), perceived partner disclosure (t = 3.27, p = 0.002) and perceived partner responsiveness (t = 3.26, p = 0.034), while their SCs had higher scores of mutual constructive communication (t = 3.70, p < 0.001), intimacy (t = 3.42, p = 0.001) and RS (t = 3.94, p < 0.001) in the IG than the CG only when these variables were low before the intervention [27]. The remaining four studies illustrated that CPs and/or their SCs obtained a greater increase in communication, intimacy, and/or RS in IG than CG only when at least one of them had communication problems (e.g., holding back) before intervention [29,30,34,36]. Notably, the offline group intervention had no any significantly different influence on couples' RS between treatment terms regardless of at post-treatment or three months follow-up [32]. Unexpectedly, Manne, et al. [27] found that the intervention may diminish level of self-disclosure of CPs, and intimacy and RS of their SCs when these variables were high before the intervention.

3.9.3. Effects on Individual Functioning for Within-Group Comparisons of Pre–Post Change

Two studies explored the effect of interventions on individual functioning in within-group comparisons of pre–post change [24,33]. One online intervention program reported that couples perceived less anxiety at follow-up periods in both the IG and the CG [24]. The other study, which focused on participants with distress before the intervention, reported that CPs and their SCs experienced an improvement in psychological distress, depression, cancer concerns and psychological adjustment during varied follow-up periods regardless of treatment arms [33].

3.9.4. Effects on Individual Functioning for Between-Group Comparisons of Pre–Post Change

Seven studies investigated the different influence of treatment arms on psychological adaptation and/or QOL. Greater improvements in post-traumatic stress, anxiety, depression and psychological adjustment at both post-treatment and six-month follow-up were reported by CPs and their SCs in the IG than the CG [26]. Moreover, Manne et al. [27] demonstrated that couples had fewer cancer-related concerns (t = -2.34, $p = 0.022$) or cancer-specific distress (t = -2.31, $p = 0.024$) in the IG than the CG, but only when these variables were high before the intervention. The offline group intervention found that CPs had more visible improvement in psychological adjustment in the two-session group than the other two treatment arms, but SCs did not [32]. In addition, Porter et al. [34] illustrated that couples seemed to gain more improvement in post-traumatic growth and self-efficacy in the CG than the IG, when the CG aimed to provide cancer-related information over six sessions [34]. Two studies that were designed to promote CPs' unidirectional self-disclosure to their SCs reported no significant change in the psychological distress of couples between treatment arms, regardless of follow-up periods [29,30]. As for QOL, CPs had a greater increase in QOL at six-month follow-up (Cohen's d = 0.48), while their SCs experienced more improvement at post-treatment (Cohen's d = 0.22) and six-month follow-up (Cohen's d = 0.31) in the IG than the CG.

4. Discussion

A total of 14 eligible articles were included in this review according to the inclusion and exclusion criteria. Through extracting and synthesizing characteristics and outcomes of these included studies, we have demonstrated the approaches and contents used in couple-based communication interventions, their feasibility and acceptability, and their effect on CP–SC dyads' psychosocial adaptation to cancer. To synoptically discuss the results of these included studies, we have arranged the construction of the Discussion section as four "Ws" (including Who, What, How, and When), efficacy, recommendations and limitations to provide some enlightenment for future research.

4.1. Who?—Choosing the Target Population

For CPs and their SCs, the diagnosis of specific types of cancer would induce specific communication needs. For example, CPs with colorectal cancer would like to communicate about ostomy-related issues and changed bowel function with their SCs [37]. There are different communication topics among couples during different cancer stages. Facing early diagnosis, CPs and their SCs may be more concerned with the treatment effect, a healthy diet and physical exercise. Meanwhile, for advanced cancer stages, there will be more difficult topics, such as making the CPs comfortable rather than cured and anticipatory grief of losing loved partners [38]. In addition, half of the articles included in this review targeted a population with gender-specific cancer (breast or prostate cancer). Gender may act as a possible factor impacting adjustment outcomes for CPs and SCs. For instance, in the context of colorectal cancer, studies reported that female CPs and female SCs usually experienced more anxiety, depression, fear of cancer recurrence [39–42] and less marital satisfaction [43] than their male counterparts. Although a systematic review and meta-analysis conducted by Hagedoorn et al. found that individual levels of distress were attributed more to gender compared with role (CP or SC) [44], focusing on participants with gender-specific cancer still makes it difficult for researchers to distinguish whether gender or role has an impact on adjustment outcomes [45]. In addition, according to intervention outcomes in this review, interventions seemed to be more beneficial for participants who experienced distress or communication problems before the intervention. Notably, one study led by Manne et al. reported that a couple-based communication intervention may reduce participants' level of self-disclosure, intimacy and RS when they had relatively high levels of relationship functioning before the intervention [27]. More research is warranted to explore whether it is necessary to assess couples' relationship or individual functioning before the intervention and select those with distress or communication problems as participants.

4.2. What?—Communication Topics

Communication topics mentioned in the included studies consisted of cancer-related experience, thoughts, feelings and relationship issues. Encouraging cancer-related emotional disclosure among CP–SC dyads is a common recommendation in couple-based interventions [46]. Badr reported that there is great variability in topics when couples talk about cancer [17]. Except for emotional disclosure, health-related topics (e.g., symptom management, treatment issues, daily care and prognosis) and relationship topics (e.g., role change, marital relationship and social/family issues) also need to be given more attention [17,47]. For example, talking about symptom management/treatment issues possibly helps couples reassert a sense of control over their cancer situation [17], talking about daily care (e.g., healthy diet and exercise) may promote couples going back to a routine life, while discussing relationship topics may activate support resources from the relationship network [11]. Therefore, it is necessary to emphasize the importance of varied topics for CP–SC dyads' psychosocial adaptation to cancer, including cancer-related emotional disclosure, healthy issues and relationship topics.

4.3. How?—Communication Methods

Teaching couples how to effectively communicate with each other was the critical content in these interventions in this review, mainly comprising of improving beneficial reciprocal self-disclosure, partner responsiveness and relationship engagement. In this review, unidirectional self-disclosure and partner responsiveness may have had limitations because it overlooked the process of SCs' self-disclosure and CPs' responsiveness. Manne et al. [48] reported that, regardless of role (CP or SC), self-disclosure and partner disclosure positively promoted the perceived partner responsiveness, and further improved their intimacy, which may be attributed to reciprocal self-disclosure and partner responsiveness being important for improving a couple's members' sense of feeling understood, validated and cared for [11]. In addition, distinguishing and declining relationship-compromising behaviors are similarly important because of their consistent association with negative outcomes [17]. As for ways of expression, except for oral discussion, this review showed that written expression was also used and was effective. With regard to communication channels, some participants regarded themselves as "face-to-face kind of person" [25], while other participants preferred using social media to communicate [47]. Therefore, it is more reasonable to provide varied communication channels to be chosen by participants.

4.4. When?—Communication Timing

With regard to intervention dosage, in general, the included studies implemented interventions in 3–4 modules/sessions (each 60–90 min in length) within six weeks, and had up to six-month-long follow-up periods. For some participants with specific situations, such as a low capability to understand, more need to communicate and disruption due to treatment, fittingly lengthening the intervention dosage is necessary. As for when to start the coupled-based communication interventions, previous studies suggested that it is better to start before some important treatment/life timepoints, such as before making a decision about treatment, surgery, the transition to survivorship and end-of-life care [11,47].

4.5. Exact Efficacy of Couple-Based Communication Interventions

Generally, the feasibility and acceptability of existing couple-based communication interventions are acceptable. The relatively low recruitment rates may not only have been due to the difficulty of conducting the psychological program, but also obstruction of recruiting CPs and their SCs simultaneously. The relatively high retention and completion rates may suggest that the interventions could greatly meet participants' communication needs, which, in turn, supports the view that it is necessary to carry out this kind of intervention to help couples adjust to cancer better. The effect sizes of interventions were identified as small (Cohen's d = 0.20–0.30), medium (Cohen's d = 0.30–0.60) and large (Cohen's d > 0.80) [26]. In this review, two studies reported small effect sizes, ranging from 0.22 to 0.30 [24,33], which were consistent with the result of a review conducted by Badr and Krebs [19]. Another two studies showed medium [34] to large effect sizes [26], ranging from 0.31 to 1.17. The relatively high effect sizes may be attributed to the clear and singular purpose of couple-based communication interventions, or the fact that they focused on participants with distress or communication problems before the intervention. It is still difficult to conclude what the reasons were for the medium to large effect sizes of interventions due to insufficient studies.

In addition, Badr, et al. suggested that researchers should move beyond a "one size fits all" approach [48,49], explore nuances of couples' communication and develop more efficacious interventions for promoting CP–SC dyads' psychosocial adaptation to cancer [17]. For example, different interactions of gender and role seem to result in varied communication performance during dyadic coping with cancer. As for female patients with male partners, male partners usually initiated cancer-related communication (e.g., treatment options), but most of them avoided communicating emotional reactions [50]. Lyons et al. [51] found that female patients experienced less depression when their male partners engaged in a lower level of protective buffering (e.g., hiding worries or waving patients' worries aside). When it came to male patients with female partners, both of them tended to deny, avoid, refuse and hold back cancer-related discussion, which may be because they wanted to protect each other, or they assumed their partner's situations, thoughts and feelings rather than assessing and resolving their partner's actual emotional problems [50]. Although male patients perceived less depression when their female partners engaged in a high level of protective buffering [51], female partners' desire to gain more emotional reaction and information from male patients needed to be given more attention [50]. According to social role theory [52], the gender difference of communication performance may be attributed to gender stereotypes, that is, men are good at instrumental behaviors while women prefer expressive behaviors. Exploring reasons or motivations for specific communication performance induced by role and gender would be helpful for researchers to better understand this specificity and provide CP–SC dyads with more personalized communication support.

4.6. Recommendations for Future Research

According to the characteristics and outcomes of intervention studies included in this review, we give the following recommendations in the hope of helping future relevant interventions:

(1) Conducted country: 93% of couple-based communication interventions were carried out in western countries, which reminds us that future interventions should be investigated in other regions, such as Asia;
(2) Target population: more research is needed to explore the necessity of screening distress or communication difficulties of CPs and/or SCs before the intervention;
(3) Study design: more longitudinal RCTs with large enough sample sizes are needed to explore the efficacy of couple-based communication interventions;
(4) Theoretical framework: a detailed combination of the theoretical framework and intervention design adopted should be reported in order to support future replicative studies;
(5) Intervention contents: focusing on varied topics, teaching couples to improve mutual communication behaviors, activating couples' relationship resources and considering specificity of gender and role during the intervention may promote the efficacy of couple-based communication interventions;
(6) Intervention delivery: to meet the CP–SC dyads' different preferences for delivery format, a combination of in-person and web-based intervention delivery is recommended to be adopted.

4.7. Limitations of this Review

It is necessary to point out that there are several limitations in this review. First, only studies published in English or Chinese were searched for and included in this review. Potential studies in other languages or published forms (e.g., conference proceedings, dissertation or editorials) may have been overlooked. Second, the heterogeneity of the included studies, such as differences in the type and stage of cancer studied, the study design, and the varied measurement tools used, may have impacted the generalization of outcomes. Third, we should be cautious to interpret the effect sizes of the interventions because they had small sample sizes and different baseline functioning. In sum, more research is needed to improve understanding and develop more efficacious couple-based communication interventions.

5. Conclusions

CP–SC dyads may experience communication difficulties while coping with cancer. Studies included in this review reported that a couple-based communication intervention improved CP–SC dyads' relationships and individual functioning, that is, to improve couples' psychosocial adaptation to cancer. More research is warranted to understand and develop more efficacious couple-based communication interventions, such as exploring the impact of the interaction of gender and role on dyads' mutual communication behaviors.

Author Contributions: Conceptualization, J.Z., X.C., Z.W. and Q.L.; methodology, J.Z. and Q.L.; validation, J.Z., X.C., Z.W. and Q.L.; formal analysis, J.Z.; investigation, J.Z., X.C. and Z.W.; resources, J.Z.; data curation, J.Z., X.C., Z.W. and Q.L.; writing—original draft preparation, J.Z.; writing—review and editing, J.Z., X.C., Z.W. and Q.L.; visualization, J.Z.; supervision, Q.L.; project administration, J.Z. and Q.L.; funding acquisition, Q.L. All authors have read and agreed to the published version of the manuscript.

Funding: This research was funded by the National Natural Science Foundation of China, grant number 82172844.

Institutional Review Board Statement: Not applicable.

Informed Consent Statement: Not applicable.

Data Availability Statement: All data used in this study are completely published online.

Conflicts of Interest: The authors declare no conflict of interest.

References

1. Sung, H.; Ferlay, J.; Siegel, R.L.; Laversanne, M.; Soerjomataram, I.; Jemal, A.; Bray, F. Global Cancer Statistics 2020: GLOBOCAN Estimates of Incidence and Mortality Worldwide for 36 Cancers in 185 Countries. *CA Cancer J. Clin.* **2021**, *71*, 209–249. [CrossRef]
2. Global Health Estimates 2020: Deaths by Cause, Age, Sex, by Country and by Region, 2000–2019. Geneva, World Health Organization. Available online: https://www.who.int/data/gho/data/themes/mortality-and-global-health-estimates/ghe-leading-causes-of-death (accessed on 31 December 2020).
3. Li, Q.; Loke, A.Y. A literature review on the mutual impact of the spousal caregiver-cancer patients dyads: 'communication', 'reciprocal influence', and 'caregiver-patient congruence'. *Eur. J. Oncol. Nurs.* **2014**, *18*, 58–65. [CrossRef]
4. Lin, Y.; Luo, X.; Li, J.; Xu, Y.; Li, Q. The dyadic relationship of benefit finding and its impact on quality of life in colorectal cancer survivor and spousal caregiver couples. *Support Care Cancer* **2021**, *29*, 1477–1486. [CrossRef]
5. Berg, C.A.; Upchurch, R. A developmental-contextual model of couples coping with chronic illness across the adult life span. *Psychol. Bull.* **2007**, *133*, 920–954. [CrossRef]
6. Li, Q.; Loke, A.Y. A preliminary conceptual framework for cancer couple dyads: Live with love. *Cancer Nurs.* **2015**, *38*, E27–E36. [CrossRef]
7. Bodenmann, G.; Falconier, M.; Randall, A.K. Systemic-Transactional Model of Dyadic Coping. In *Encyclopedia of Couple and Family Therapy*; Springer International Publishing AG: Berlin, Germany, 2017. [CrossRef]
8. Kayser, K.; Msw, L.E.W.; Msw, L.T.A. Cancer as a "we-disease": Examining the process of coping from a relational perspective. *Fam. Syst. Health* **2007**, *4*, 404–418. [CrossRef]
9. Badr, H.; Milbury, K.; Majeed, N.; Carmack, C.L.; Ahmad, Z.; Gritz, E.R. Natural language use and couples' adjustment to head and neck cancer. *Health Psychol.* **2016**, *35*, 1069–1080. [CrossRef]
10. Donovan, E.E.; LeBlanc, F.K. Interpersonal Communication and Coping with Cancer: A Multidisciplinary Theoretical Review of the Literature: CT. *Commun. Theory* **2019**, *29*, 236–256. [CrossRef]
11. Manne, S.; Badr, H. Intimacy and relationship processes in couples' psychosocial adaptation to cancer. *Cancer* **2008**, *112*, 2541–2555. [CrossRef]
12. Chen, M.; Gong, J.; Cao, Q.; Luo, X.; Li, J.; Li, Q. A literature review of the relationship between dyadic coping and dyadic outcomes in cancer couples. *Eur. J. Oncol. Nurs.* **2021**, *54*, 102035. [CrossRef]
13. Manne, S.; Badr, H.; Zaider, T.; Nelson, C.; Kissane, D. Cancer-related communication, relationship intimacy, and psychological distress among couples coping with localized prostate cancer. *J. Cancer Surviv.* **2010**, *4*, 74–85. [CrossRef] [PubMed]
14. Manne, S.L.; Kissane, D.; Zaider, T.; Kashy, D.; Lee, D.; Heckman, C.; Virtue, S.M. Holding back, intimacy, and psychological and relationship outcomes among couples coping with prostate cancer. *J. Fam. Psychol.* **2015**, *29*, 708–719. [CrossRef] [PubMed]
15. Li, Q.; Loke, A.Y. A systematic review of spousal couple-based intervention studies for couples coping with cancer: Direction for the development of interventions. *Psychooncology* **2014**, *23*, 731–739. [CrossRef] [PubMed]
16. Luo, X.; Li, J.; Chen, M.; Gong, J.; Xu, Y.; Li, Q. A literature review of post-treatment survivorship interventions for colorectal cancer survivors and/or their caregivers. *Psychooncology* **2021**, *30*, 807–817. [CrossRef]
17. Badr, H. New frontiers in couple-based interventions in cancer care: Refining the prescription for spousal communication. *Acta Oncol.* **2017**, *56*, 139–145. [CrossRef] [PubMed]
18. Helgeson, V.S.; Jakubiak, B.K.; Van Vleet, M.; Zajdel, M. Communal Coping and Adjustment to Chronic Illness: Theory Update and Evidence. *Pers. Soc. Psychol. Rev.* **2018**, *22*, 170–195. [CrossRef] [PubMed]
19. Badr, H.; Krebs, P. A systematic review and meta-analysis of psychosocial interventions for couples coping with cancer. *Psychooncology* **2013**, *22*, 1688–1704. [CrossRef]
20. Lu, X. The Development and Evalution of a WeChat-Based Couples Coping Focused Supportive Intervention for Couples Coping with Colorectal Cancer as Dyads. Master's Thesis, Jiangnan University, Wuxi, China, 2021.
21. Armijo-Olivo, S.; Stiles, C.R.; Hagen, N.A.; Biondo, P.D.; Cummings, G.G. Assessment of study quality for systematic reviews: A comparison of the Cochrane Collaboration Risk of Bias Tool and the Effective Public Health Practice Project Quality Assessment Tool: Methodological research. *J. Eval. Clin. Pract.* **2012**, *18*, 12–18. [CrossRef]
22. Thomas, B.H.; Ciliska, D.; Dobbins, M.; Micucci, S. A process for systematically reviewing the literature: Providing the research evidence for public health nursing interventions. *Worldviews Evid. Based Nurs.* **2004**, *1*, 176–184. [CrossRef]
23. Fergus, K.D.; McLeod, D.; Carter, W.; Warner, E.; Gardner, S.L.; Granek, L.; Cullen, K.I. Development and pilot testing of an online intervention to support young couples' coping and adjustment to breast cancer. *Eur. J. Cancer Care* **2014**, *23*, 481–492. [CrossRef]
24. Fergus, K.; Ahmad, S.; Gardner, S.; Ianakieva, I.; McLeod, D.; Stephen, J.; Carter, W.; Periera, A.; Warner, E.; Panchaud, J. Couplelinks online intervention for young couples facing breast cancer: A randomised controlled trial. *Psychooncology* **2022**, *31*, 512–520. [CrossRef]
25. Fergus, K.; Tanen, A.; Ahmad, S.; Gardner, S.; Warner, E.; McLeod, D.; Stephen, J.; Carter, W.; Periera, A. Treatment Satisfaction with Couplelinks Online Intervention to Promote Dyadic Coping in Young Couples Affected by Breast Cancer. *Front. Psychol.* **2022**, *13*, 862555. [CrossRef]

26. Gremore, T.M.; Brockstein, B.; Porter, L.S.; Brenner, S.; Benfield, T.; Baucom, D.H.; Sher, T.G.; Atkins, D. Couple-based communication intervention for head and neck cancer: A randomized pilot trial. *Support. Care Cancer Off. J. Multinatl. Assoc. Support. Care Cancer* **2020**, *29*, 3267–3275. [CrossRef] [PubMed]
27. Manne, S.L.; Kissane, D.W.; Nelson, C.J.; Mulhall, J.P.; Winkel, G.; Zaider, T. Intimacy-enhancing psychological intervention for men diagnosed with prostate cancer and their partners: A pilot study. *J. Sex Med.* **2011**, *8*, 1197–1209. [CrossRef]
28. Mowll, J.; Lobb, E.A.; Lane, L.; Lacey, J.; Chochinov, H.M.; Kelly, B.; Agar, M.; Links, M.; Kearsley, J.H. A preliminary study to develop an intervention to facilitate communication between couples in advanced cancer. *Palliat. Support. Care* **2015**, *13*, 1381–1390. [CrossRef] [PubMed]
29. Porter, L.S.; Keefe, F.J.; Baucom, D.H.; Hurwitz, H.; Moser, B.; Patterson, E.; Kim, H.J. Partner-assisted emotional disclosure for patients with gastrointestinal cancer: Results from a randomized controlled trial. *Cancer* **2009**, *115*, 4326–4338. [CrossRef] [PubMed]
30. Porter, L.S.; Keefe, F.J.; Baucom, D.H.; Hurwitz, H.; Moser, B.; Patterson, E.; Kim, H.J. Partner-assisted emotional disclosure for patients with GI cancer: 8-week follow-up and processes associated with change. *Support. Care Cancer* **2012**, *20*, 1755–1762. [CrossRef]
31. Porter, L.S.; Baucom, D.H.; Keefe, F.J.; Patterson, E.S. Reactions to a partner-assisted emotional disclosure intervention: Direct observation and self-report of patient and partner communication. *J. Marital. Fam. Ther.* **2012**, *38*, 284–295. [CrossRef]
32. Shields, C.G.; Rousseau, S.J. A pilot study of an intervention for breast cancer survivors and their spouses. *Fam. Process* **2004**, *43*, 95–107. [CrossRef]
33. Manne, S.L.; Kashy, D.A.; Zaider, T.; Kissane, D.; Lee, D.; Kim, I.Y.; Heckman, C.J.; Penedo, F.J.; Murphy, E.; Virtue, S.M. Couple-focused interventions for men with localized prostate cancer and their spouses: A randomized clinical trial. *Br. J. Health Psychol.* **2019**, *24*, 396–418. [CrossRef]
34. Porter, L.S.; Keefe, F.J.; Baucom, D.H.; Olsen, M.; Zafar, S.Y.; Uronis, H. A randomized pilot trial of a videoconference couples communication intervention for advanced GI cancer. *Psycho-Oncology* **2017**, *26*, 1027–1035. [CrossRef] [PubMed]
35. Porter, L.S.; Fish, L.; Steinhauser, K. Themes Addressed by Couples with Advanced Cancer during a Communication Skills Training Intervention. *J. Pain Symptom Manag.* **2018**, *56*, 252–258. [CrossRef] [PubMed]
36. Su, S.; Zheng, W.; Liu, M.; Kang, T.; Wang, D.; Liu, H. Application of Couples Communication Skills Training in Patients with Advanced Gastric Cancer and Their Spouse. *Nurs. J. Chin. PLA* **2022**, *39*, 14–17. [CrossRef]
37. Cheng, X.; Du, R.; Zhou, H.; Chen, C.; Li, Y.; Wang, T. Disease communication experience between couples in patients with colorectal cancer stoma: A qualitative study. *Chin. J. Nurs.* **2021**, *56*, 721–726.
38. McLean, L.M.; Jones, J.M. A review of distress and its management in couples facing end-of-life cancer. *Psychooncology* **2007**, *16*, 603–616. [CrossRef]
39. Akyol, M.; Ulger, E.; Alacacioglu, A.; Kucukzeybek, Y.; Yildiz, Y.; Bayoglu, V.; Gumus, Z.; Yildiz, I.; Salman, T.; Varol, U.; et al. Sexual satisfaction, anxiety, depression and quality of life among Turkish colorectal cancer patients [Izmir Oncology Group (IZOG) study]. *Jpn. J. Clin. Oncol.* **2015**, *45*, 657–664. [CrossRef]
40. Zhou, L.; Sun, H. The longitudinal changes of anxiety and depression, their related risk factors and prognostic value in colorectal cancer survivors: A 36-month follow-up study. *Clin. Res. Hepatol. Gastroenterol.* **2021**, *45*, 101511. [CrossRef]
41. Tuinstra, J.; Hagedoorn, M.; Van Sonderen, E.; Ranchor, A.V.; Van den Bos, G.A.; Nijboer, C.; Sanderman, R. Psychological distress in couples dealing with colorectal cancer: Gender and role differences and intracouple correspondence. *Br. J. Health Psychol.* **2004**, *9*, 465–478. [CrossRef]
42. Northouse, L.L.; Mood, D.; Templin, T.; Mellon, S.; George, T. Couples' patterns of adjustment to colon cancer. *Soc. Sci. Med.* **2000**, *50*, 271–284. [CrossRef]
43. Kayser, K.; Acquati, C.; Reese, J.B.; Mark, K.; Wittmann, D.; Karam, E. A systematic review of dyadic studies examining relationship quality in couples facing colorectal cancer together. *Psychooncology* **2018**, *27*, 13–21. [CrossRef] [PubMed]
44. Hagedoorn, M.; Sanderman, R.; Bolks, H.N.; Tuinstra, J.; Coyne, J.C. Distress in couples coping with cancer: A meta-analysis and critical review of role and gender effects. *Psychol. Bull.* **2008**, *134*, 1–30. [CrossRef] [PubMed]
45. Kim, Y.; Mitchell, H.R.; Ting, A. Application of psychological theories on the role of gender in caregiving to psycho-oncology research. *Psychooncology* **2019**, *28*, 228–254. [CrossRef] [PubMed]
46. Badr, H. Author's response to Porter and Keefe letter to the editor regarding 'new frontiers in couple-based interventions in cancer care: Refining the prescription for spousal communication'. *Acta Oncol.* **2018**, *57*, 695–697. [CrossRef]
47. Li, J.; Luo, X.; Cao, Q.; Lin, Y.; Xu, Y.; Li, Q. Communication Needs of Cancer Patients and/or Caregivers: A Critical Literature Review. *J. Oncol.* **2020**, *2020*, 7432849. [CrossRef] [PubMed]
48. Manne, S.; Ostroff, J.; Rini, C.; Fox, K.; Goldstein, L.; Grana, G. The interpersonal process model of intimacy: The role of self-disclosure, partner disclosure, and partner responsiveness in interactions between breast cancer patients and their partners. *J. Fam. Psychol.* **2004**, *18*, 589–599. [CrossRef] [PubMed]
49. Porter, L.S.; Keefe, F.J. Couple-based communication interventions for cancer: Moving beyond a 'one size fits all' approach. *Acta Oncol.* **2018**, *57*, 693–695. [CrossRef] [PubMed]
50. Lim, J.W.; Paek, M.S.; Shon, E.J. Gender and Role Differences in Couples' Communication during Cancer Survivorship. *Cancer Nurs.* **2015**, *38*, E51–E60. [CrossRef]

51. Lyons, K.S.; Gorman, J.R.; Larkin, B.S.; Duncan, G.; Hayes-Lattin, B. Active Engagement, Protective Buffering, and Depressive Symptoms in Young-Midlife Couples Surviving Cancer: The Roles of Age and Sex. *Front. Psychol.* **2022**, *13*, 816626. [CrossRef]
52. Eagly, A.H.; Wood, W. Social role theory. In *Handbook of Theories of Social Psychology*; Van Lange, P.A.M., Kruglanski, A.W., Eds.; SAGE Publications Ltd.: London, UK, 2012; Volume 2, pp. 458–476.

Disclaimer/Publisher's Note: The statements, opinions and data contained in all publications are solely those of the individual author(s) and contributor(s) and not of MDPI and/or the editor(s). MDPI and/or the editor(s) disclaim responsibility for any injury to people or property resulting from any ideas, methods, instructions or products referred to in the content.

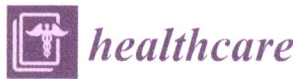

Article

The Role of Resilience in the Relationship between Sociodemographic, Clinical Characteristics, and Social Support among Breast Cancer Patients in Serbia

Sanja D Tomić [1,*], Goran Malenković [1], Armin Šljivo [2], Ermina Mujičić [2] and Slobodan Tomić [1]

1 Faculty of Medicine, University of Novi Sad, 21000 Novi Sad, Serbia; goran.malenkovic@mf.uns.ac.rs (G.M.); 907002d21@mf.uns.ac.rs (S.T.)
2 Clinical Center, University of Sarajevo, 71000 Sarajevo, Bosnia and Herzegovina; sljivo95@windowslive.com (A.Š.); ermina.mujicic@fzs.unsa.ba (E.M.)
* Correspondence: sanja.tomic@mf.uns.ac.rs

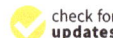

Citation: Tomić, S.D.; Malenković, G.; Šljivo, A.; Mujičić, E.; Tomić, S. The Role of Resilience in the Relationship between Sociodemographic, Clinical Characteristics, and Social Support among Breast Cancer Patients in Serbia. *Healthcare* **2023**, *11*, 3184. https://doi.org/10.3390/healthcare11243184

Academic Editor: Qiuping Li

Received: 26 October 2023
Revised: 13 December 2023
Accepted: 14 December 2023
Published: 16 December 2023

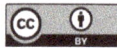

Copyright: © 2023 by the authors. Licensee MDPI, Basel, Switzerland. This article is an open access article distributed under the terms and conditions of the Creative Commons Attribution (CC BY) license (https://creativecommons.org/licenses/by/4.0/).

Abstract: Background. The management of breast cancer treatments within the limitations of family, social, and professional life is emotionally burdening and negatively affects physical, psychological, and social well-being, reducing the overall quality of life of patients and their families. Methods: This cross-sectional descriptive–analytical study was conducted from March to August 2023 at the "Dr. Radivoj Simonović" General Hospital in Sombor. A total of 236 breast cancer patients participated in this study. The research was conducted using the following instruments: a questionnaire on sociodemographic and clinical characteristics of patients, the Berlin Social-Support Scales—for assessing social support—and the Connor–Davidson Resilience Scale—for assessing resilience. This study aimed to determine the predictors and levels of social support and resilience of breast cancer patients. We also wanted to examine whether resilience is a mediator between patients' sociodemographic and clinical characteristics and levels of social support. Results: The total average value of social support was 3.51 ± 0.63, while on the resilience scale, the respondents achieved a total average score of 52.2 ± 9.63. Perceived and actually received social support of breast cancer patients were positively correlated with resilience [$p < 0.01$], while no statistically significant correlations were found for the need for support and satisfaction. The sets of predictors can significantly predict their effects on all types of perceived social support (emotional social support: 9%; perceived instrumental social support: 9%) and all types of received social support (actually received emotional social support: 8%; actually received instrumental social support: 7%; actually received informational social support: 8%). There is a potential mediating role of resilience in relation to sociodemographic factors, clinical characteristics, and the need for support. Conclusion: This study confirms that a strong connection exists between social support and resilience. However, the analysis did not confirm the mediating role of resilience between the sociodemographic and clinical characteristics on the one hand and social support on the other.

Keywords: breast cancer; Serbia; resilience; affective well-being; support

1. Introduction

The incidence and prevalence of breast cancer are constantly increasing; women all over the world most often face this particular diagnosis [1,2]. However, the number of breast cancer survivors is also increasing [3]. Coping with breast cancer, medical treatment protocols, the experience and life within the family, social, and professional contexts with all the limitations imposed by the disease, and its treatment can be upsetting and hard for patients and their families. The challenges that patients face involve a full range of negative effects on physical, psychological, and social functioning, resulting in the reduced quality of these patients' lives [4–7]; this has encouraged many authors to search for factors that influence life after treatment [8–11]. As one of those factors, social support has been discussed as a valuable resource that mitigates the effects of stressful life events on health. It has consistently been associated with better mental health, self-esteem, physical health, and longevity [12].

Social support definitions state that it refers to the quality of supportive interactions a person has with other individuals and can play a significant role in well-being [13]. Social support is thought to function as a buffer to protect individuals from the physical and mental effects of stress [14]. As defined by the National Cancer Institute (NCI), social support is a network of family members, friends, neighbors, and community members who are available in times of need to provide psychological, physical, and financial assistance to cancer patients [15]. Cohen et al. state that adequate social support should meet the needs of patients and enable the development of an optimal method of coping with the disease because excessive support in a person's life can negatively impact their activity and lead to the loss of independence [12].

There are several theoretical frameworks that explain the multidimensional effects of social support on the well-being and health of adults. The most widely accepted are the buffering and direct effect models. The first suggests that support reduces the harm of stressful events by preventing the individual from considering the situation as threatening or demanding [14]. On the other hand, the direct effect model suggests that social support is beneficial regardless of the amount of stress an individual perceives. In this model, the understanding that others are willing to help increases self-esteem and provides the individual with a sense of control over their situation [12].

Belonging to a social network can directly influence treatment outcomes by positively influencing treatment adherence and disease management [8]. An individual's social network is essential to fully participate in and benefit from all facets of cancer treatment, including symptom management, care coordination, assistance with daily activities, and emotional support [16]. Despite the lack of consensus regarding the definition of social support, most authors emphasize the importance of perceived and actually received support [16–19]. Perceived social support refers to the expected availability of support in the future, whereas actual social support refers to the actual experiences of individuals. Furthermore, according to the type of support provided, it is possible to distinguish between instrumental, informational, and emotional support [12]. Emotional support is the care and support that inspires trust and a sense of belonging and love. Instrumental support is helping with practical tasks, such as transportation, childcare, and financial assistance. Informational support consists of knowledge, information, and advice [18]. For the purposes of this study, the above-mentioned concept was applied. These definitions take into account important aspects of this concept, i.e., the level of support received from diverse sources and the degree of satisfaction of individuals with this support, thus increasing resilience and giving individuals the courage to face challenges, improving their own adaptability and quality of life.

There is a general agreement among researchers that the disease usually limits patients' participation in social activities, implicating that the opportunities to interact with others and their access to social support may be reduced [11–14]. Alternatively, the patients themselves may choose to withdraw from their social network. In both cases, this is related to a patient's cancer experience, which depends on variables such as demographic (age, gender, socioeconomic status, etc.) and clinical (site of malignancy, stage of disease, and type of treatment) characteristics [11,15]. The results confirm that effective ways of coping with stress are significantly lower in women who have completed primary school and who have not undergone surgery. The levels of effective coping with stress in women subsides with increasing age, and as the perceived score of social support increases, so does the level of effective coping with stress. Findings show that social support and age significantly predict effective stress management [20]. In addition, negative relationships are found between the level of resilience and the time of diagnosis. Regarding the different treatments administered to the patients, experience with chemotherapy is the factor that produced the greatest impact in terms of increasing the level of resilience [21]. Previous studies indicate that one-quarter to one-third of breast cancer patients will develop anxiety and/or depression at some point during their treatment [20], and those under 50 are particularly likely to report psychological distress [22,23]. Psychological resistance, or resilience, can be defined as an individual's ability to maintain or restore relatively stable psychological and physical functioning during or after significant stressful life events [24]. In cancer patients, resilience refers to a dynamic process that promotes successful adaptation to cancer-related hardships [25]. The relationship between resilience and social support in the cancer survivor population has already been established in some studies [26]. An Indian study shows that being optimistic not only attracts others but also encourages the establishment of social support networks. Moreover, optimism and social support play a vital role in improving the general well-being of cancer patients. Also, belonging to social networks has a direct impact on the treatment outcomes and is effective regarding the perceived vs. actually received social support and considering their distinct types, such as emotional, instrumental, and informational. Although a cancer diagnosis involves personal suffering, many women with breast cancer can develop the ability to resist and accept life's crises, resulting in greater resilience.

Therefore, this study aimed to determine the levels of social support and resilience of breast cancer patients. We also wanted to examine the effects of predictors on the levels of social support and whether resilience was a mediator between patients' sociodemographic and clinical characteristics and levels of social support.

2. Materials and Methods

This descriptive–analytical cross-sectional study was conducted from March to August 2023. The sample consisted of patients at the 'Dr. Radivoj Simonović' General Hospital in Sombor. All adult patients diagnosed with breast cancer took part in the research. Inclusion criteria were (1) diagnosis of breast cancer in women from stage 0 to stage IV; (2) completed cancer treatment, i.e., chemotherapy, hormone therapy, targeted therapy, immunotherapy, treatment of bone metastases, or any combination of these; and (3) the ability to communicate in the Serbian language. Participation in this study was voluntary and anonymous, with previously signed written consent from the participants. Exclusion criteria were any psychiatric or addictive disorders.

2.1. Research Instruments

Three Instruments Were Used in the Planned Research
Berlin Social-Support Scales [BSSS]

This is a set of self-report questionnaires developed by Schultz and Schwarzer [18] to assess social support. The BSSS includes six individual domains: perceived available support (8 items), need for support (4 items), support seeking (5 items), actually received social support (14 items), protective buffering (6 items), and satisfaction (1 item). The total number of BSSS items is 38. Using a multidimensional approach to measurement in the domain of perceived social support, it is possible to distinguish between two types of perceived social support, namely perceived emotional social support and perceived instrumental social support. Also, in the domain of actually received social support, three types are distinguished: actually received emotional social support, actually received instrumental social support, and actually received informational social support. The scale was validated on the sample of adult cancer patients with Cronbach's alpha coefficients (a) ranging from 0.75 to 0.96 [18]. The response format for participants was consistent across domains. Participants rated their agreement with the statements on the BSSS scale as follows: strongly disagree (1), somewhat disagree (2), somewhat agree (3), and strongly agree (4). A higher score reflects a higher level of social support.

Connor–Davidson Resilience Scale [CD-RISC-25]

The CD-RISC-25 consists of statements that describe several aspects of resilience. The scale includes 25 items that measure resilience in 6 subscales: hardiness, coping, adaptability/flexibility, meaningfulness, optimism, and self-efficacy. Each item is scored from 0 to 4. A total score is obtained by summing all 25 items, giving a score that can range from 0 to 100. Lower scores indicate less resilience, and higher scores indicate greater resilience.

Sociodemographic Questionnaire and Clinical Characteristics of the Participants

The sociodemographic questionnaire for collecting data relevant to this study includes questions regarding the following: age, gender, educational attainment, employment, place of residence, socioeconomic status, and partner status. Socioeconomic status was assessed based on participants' income. In relation to the amount of monthly income, they are classified into three categories. Average socioeconomic status is defined by income from EUR 600 to 1000; below the average is anything less than EUR 600, and above the average is anything greater than EUR 1000.

The clinical variables questionnaire to collect data relevant to this study included questions regarding the following: the time passed since cancer treatment, treatment modalities, fatigue, pain, and the presence of stress in the past year. Fatigue is defined as a feeling of physical exhaustion and lack of energy, and it is measured numerically by assessing its intensity at the time of the survey. Participants were asked to indicate the number on the NRS that best represented their current level of fatigue ("How tired are you feeling right now?") using a 10-point fatigue scale (0 = "no fatigue"; 10 = "worst possible fatigue"). A 10-point fatigue scale has been well-validated to assess fatigue in people with cancer [27,28]. For the purposes of this study, fatigue was classified as follows: grades 0–3—no fatigue; 4–6—mild fatigue; and 7–10—intense fatigue. A visual analog scale was used to assess pain at the time of the survey. It was a 10 cm long numerical scale divided into 10 parts with three verbal descriptors. No scale was used to reassess stress, but participants were asked to clarify whether or not they had experienced stress during the last year.

2.2. Statistical Data Processing

Statistical analysis was performed using SPSS Statistics software (IBM SPSS Statistics for Windows, Version 22.0, Armonk, NY, USA). The results were tabulated, showing descriptive statistics data (frequencies and percentages for categorical data, as well as arithmetic means and standard deviations for quantitative data). The impact of patients' sociodemographic and clinical characteristics on certain types of social support was calculated using the *t*-test and one-way analysis of variance (ANOVA). Correlations of social support and resilience were calculated using the Pearson correlation coefficient. Predictive variables consisted of sociodemographic characteristics in the first step, clinical characteristics in the second step, and dimensions of resilience in the third step of the hierarchical regression analysis. Considering significant predictor variables and their effects, a series of multiple regression analyses were conducted with social support (perceived and actual) as outcome variables. Cronbach's Alpha reliability coefficient was used to assess the reliability of the instruments used.

2.3. Ethical Consent

In addition to the consent of the authors of the questionnaire, the consent of the Ethics Committee of the Faculty of Medicine in Novi Sad (Decision no. 01-39/34/1/2023) and the consent of the Ethics Committee of the General Hospital "Dr. Radivoj Simonović" in Sombor were obtained for conducting the research and using the research instruments (Decision No: 23-3108/2023).

3. Results

A total of 236 female participants took part in this study, with the highest percentage of women over 51 years old (65.7%). The majority (55.1%) completed primary education. About half of the participants (50.8%) were unemployed, and 61% lived in urban areas.

In addition, 71.2% reported having a partner, and 50.8% rated their socioeconomic status as average. The treatment for the majority of participants was completed in the last 3 years (64.4%), and in the last year, half of them stated that they had no stress. Combined treatment, which includes both local and systemic methods, was administered to 67.8% of study participants. Almost half of the study participants (49.2% vs. 45.8%) experienced mild pain and fatigue. All other data regarding age, education, professional activity, place of residence, socioeconomic status, partners, and clinical variables in patients with breast cancer are shown in Table 1.

Table 1. Sociodemographic and clinical characteristics.

Sociodemographic Variables	%	N
Age (years)		
≤50	34.3	81
≥51	65.7	155
Education		
Other than college	55.1	130
College/University	44.9	106
Professional activity		
Active	49.2	116
Inactive	50.8	120
Residence		
Rural	39.0	92
Urban	61.0	144
Self—reported financial standing		
Below average	33.5	79
Average	50.8	120
Above average	15.7	37
Partner		
Yes	71.2	168
No	28.8	68
Clinical variables	%	N
Stress		
Yes	47.5	112
No	52.1	123
Time since treatment (years)		
≤1	22.9	54
>1–≤3	41.5	98
>3	35.6	84
Type of treatment		
Only local therapy	25.4	60
Systemic therapy	6.8	16
Combined therapy	67.8	160
The pain		
Without pain	38.1	90
Mild	49.2	116
Strong	12.7	30
The fatigue		
Non-existent	17.8	42
Mild	45.8	108
Intense	36.4	86

3.1. Descriptive Statistics and Correlation Coefficients CD-RISC-25 and BSSS

Table 2 shows the average scores for CD-RISC-25 and BSSS for the entire sample. CD-RISC-25 ranges from 0 to 100, with an average total score of 52.2 (SD = 9.63). The average total score for BSSS was 3.51 (SD = 0.63) out of 4.

Table 2. Average scores on CD-RISC-25 and BSSS scales.

	Total Range Min–Max	Total Mean (SD)
CD-RISC-25	0–100	52.2 (9.63)
BSSS	0–4	3.51 (0.63)

Considering the correlation of resilience and social support, significant correlations were recorded with the intensity ranging from 0.255 to 0.487, all of which were positive. These results show that higher resilience is directly connected with higher social support. Resilience does correlate with the domains 'need for support' and 'satisfaction', but these correlations are not statistically significant (Table 3).

Table 3. Correlation of social support and resilience.

	PESS	PISS	NS	SS	SATIS	ARES	ARInsS	ARInfS	CD-RISC-25
PESS	1								
PISS	0.535 **	1							
NS	0.262 **	0.356 **	1						
SS	0.129	0.373 **	0.490 **	1					
SATIS	0.052	0.059	0.047	−0.005	1				
ARES	0.293 **	0.406 **	0.173	0.275 **	0.145	1			
ARInsS	0.465 **	0.469 **	0.294 **	0.262 **	0.123	0.436 **	1		
ARInfS	0.331 **	0.344 **	0.247 **	0.302 **	0.127	0.371 **	0.374 **	1	
CD-RISC-25	0.487 **	0.469 **	0.182	0.255 **	0.106	0.371 **	0.418 **	0.337 **	1

** $p < 0.01$. PESS—perceived emotional social support; PISS—perceived instrumental social support; NS—need of support; SS—seeking support; SATIS—satisfaction; ARES—actual received emotional social support; ARInsS—actual received instrumental social support; ARInfS—actual received information social support.

3.2. Effects of Sociodemographic and Clinical Variables on the Types of Social Support

The results showed that participants older than 50 were more inclined to seek support from others and protect their environment from information and diagnoses related to diseases. Participants with lower educational qualifications had a greater need for support and a higher level of support seeking, while employed participants protected their social environment more from illness and diagnosis information (Table 4).

Regarding other sociodemographic variables, there were no statistically significant differences in BSSS domains based on whether they lived in a rural or urban area, had a partner, and had socioeconomic status. Participants who underwent systemic therapy showed higher levels of support seeking and higher satisfaction with support. Regarding pain, it was observed that participants who reported no pain had significantly higher perceived instrumental and emotional support compared to those with mild to severe pain. In the domain of actually received social support, pain-free patients generally experienced more actually received emotional, instrumental, and informational social support. The effects of fatigue showed that it exists, but only in the domain of perceived social support and that it did not affect the actual received social support. Patients without fatigue perceived significantly higher perceived emotional and perceived instrumental social support and were more inclined to seek support. No statistically significant differences were observed between the remaining two groups of patients categorized according to fatigue ($p > 0.05$). Participants without stress reported significantly lower support-seeking compared to those who were stressed (Table 4).

Table 4. Effects of sociodemographic and clinical variables on types of social support.

Types of Social Support	Sociodemographic Variables	Mean ± SD	Statistic Test/p
Seeking support	Age (years) ≤50 years ≥51 years	2.65 ± 0.83 2.95 ± 0.66	t = −2.34/0.03
	Education Primary/High school Bachelor	2.91 ± 0.78 2.60 ± 0.75	T = 2.24/0.03
Protective buffering support	Age (years) ≤50 ≥51	2.49 ± 0.76 2.71 ± 0.65	t = −2.05/0.05
	Professional activity Active Inactive	2.78 ± 0.78 2.39 ± 0.69	t = 2.08/0.04
Need for support	Education Primary/High school Bachelor	2.95 ± 0.62 2.64 ± 0.64	t = 2.68/0.01
	Clinical variables	**Mean ± SD**	**Statistic test/p**
Need for support	Type of treatment Only local therapy Systemic therapy Combined therapy	2.62 ± 0.92 3.20 ± 0.51 2.73 ± 0.75	F = 3.78/0.03
	Stress Yes No	3.03 ± 1.02 2.71 ± 0.82	t = 1.94/0.05
Satisfaction	Fatigue Non-existent Mild Intense	3.04 ± 0.99 2.32 ± 0.68 2.89 ± 0.80	F = 6.90/0.00
	Pain Without the pain Mild Strong	3.67 ± 0.99 3.16 ± 0.68 2.75 ± 0.80	F = 7.53/0.00
	Type of treatment Only local therapy Systemic therapy Combined therapy	3.04 ± 0.99 3.60 ± 0.68 3.46 ± 0.80	F = 3.33/0.04
Perceived instrumental social support	Time since treatment (years) ≤1 >1–≤3 >3	3.48 ± 0.71 3.01 ± 0.90 3.12 ± 0.77	F = 3.17/0.05
	Pain Without the pain Mild Strong	3.38 ± 0.93 3.08 ± 0.52 2.56 ± 0.80	F = 3.59/0.03
	Fatigue Non-existent Mild Intense	3.58 ± 0.93 2.81 ± 0.52 3.26 ± 0.80	F = 5.19/0.01

Table 4. Cont.

Types of Social Support	Sociodemographic Variables	Mean ± SD	Statistic Test/p
Perceived emotional social support	Pain Without the pain Mild Strong	3.45 ± 0.49 3.06 ± 0.78 2.81 ± 0.99	F = 6.14/0.00
	Fatigue Non-existent Mild Intense	3.64 ± 0.36 3.00 ± 0.80 3.26 ± 0.67	F = 3.90/0.02
Actual received emotional social support	Pain Without the pain Mild Strong	3.18 ± 0.41 2.90 ± 0.58 2.71 ± 0.63	F = 5.62/0.01
Actual received instrumental social support	Pain Without the pain Mild Strong	3.55 ± 0.93 3.15 ± 0.52 2.92 ± 0.80	F = 4.77/0.01
Actual received information social support	Pain Without the pain Mild Strong	3.34 ± 0.97 2.84 ± 0.77 2.87 ± 0.84	F = 5.84/0.00

3.3. Social Support Predictors

Having taken into account the significant predictor variables and their effects in the earlier stage of the analysis, a set of multiple regression analyses were conducted with social support (perceived and actually received) as the dependent variable (Table 5).

Table 5. Predictors of social support.

	PESS F = 6.36, df = 2123, $p < 0.001$, $R^2 = 0.09$		PISS F = 3.84, df = 3120, $p < 0.005$, $R^2 = 0.09$		ARES F = 11.20, df = 1124, $p < 0.001$, $R^2 = 0.08$		ARInsS F = 9.45, df = 1126, $p < 0.001$, $R^2 = 0.07$		ARInfS F = 10.40, df = 1127, $p < 0.001$, $R^2 = 0.08$	
	β	t	β	t	β	t	β	t	β	t
Age	-	-	-	-	-	-	-	-	-	-
Education	-	-	-	-	-	-	-	-	-	-
Time since treatment	-	-	−0.19	−2.11 *	-	-	-	-	-	-
Pain	−0.29	−3.37 **	−0.24	−2.67 **	−0.29	−3.35 **	−0.26	−3.07 **	−0.28	−3.32 **
Fatigue	−0.06	−0.73	−0.03	−0.36						
Stress	-	-	-	-	-	-	-	-	-	-
Professional activity	-	-	-	-	-	-	-	-	-	-

** $p < 0.01$, * $p < 0.05$. PESS—perceived emotional social support; PISS—perceived instrumental social support; ARES—actual received emotional social support; ARInsS—actual received instrumental social support; ARInfS—actual received information social support.

By looking at the results of a set of multiple regression analyses, it can be concluded that sets of predictors can significantly predict their effects on perceived emotional social support (9%), perceived instrumental social support (9%), actual emotional support (8%), actual instrumental support (7%), and actual informational support (8%).

3.4. Resilience as a Mediator in the Relationship between Patients' Sociodemographic and Clinical Characteristics and Social Support

In order to verify whether resilience is a mediator between sociodemographic and clinical characteristics of patients and social support, a hierarchical multiple regression analysis was conducted (Tables 6–8). The results of the hierarchical analysis are presented only for the types of social support where we have identified the mediating role of resilience. For domains of social support as dependent variables, sociodemographic characteristics were entered in the first step of the hierarchical multiple regression analysis, clinical characteristics in the second step, and resilience aspects (Connor–Davidson Resilience Scale CD-RISC-25) in the third step.

The results indicate that greater adaptability, better emotional–cognitive regulation, and a lower level of searching for meaning in patients potentially lead to a greater need for support at the expense of age, socioeconomic status, and level of education. In particular, the effects of these three sociodemographic variables on the need for support decrease when resilience dimensions are considered, but their effects remain significant. This model explains 25% of the variance in support seeking via the predictor variables.

A significant contribution to perceived instrumental support is only provided by the level of education. In this model, perceived instrumental support is determined by the set of predictor variables to the extent of 20%.

There is no mediating role of resilience in the relationship between the time elapsed since treatment and actual received emotional social support. However, after introducing resilience, the results indicate that actual received emotional social support will be provided to more resilient patients. In this way, 32% of actual received emotional social support is explained.

Table 6. Mediator effect of sociodemographic, clinical characteristics, and resilience to the expression of support needs.

	Step 1 $F = 3.70$, $p = 0.001$, $R^2 = 0.13$		Step 2 $F = 2.70, p = 0.015$, $R^2 = 0.15, \Delta R^2 = 0.02$, $p = 0.767$		Step 3 $F = 2.77, p = 0.001$, $R^2 = 0.25, \Delta R^2 = 0.12$, $p = 0.005$	
	β	t	β	t	β	t
Age	−0.246	−2.579 *	−0.259	−2.225 *	−0.226	−2.709
Education	−0.436	−4.174 *	−0.450	−3.995 *	−0.428	−4.484 *
Professional activity	0.220	2.190 *	0.168	1.556	0.015	0.138
Residence	−0.046	−0.441	−0.071	−0.632	0.080	0.694
Self-reported financial standing	0.319	3.110 *	0.328	3.114 *	0.271	2.666
Partner	−0.029	−0.277	−0.055	−0.507	−0.092	−0.889
Stress	-	-	0.106	1.029	0.097	0.994
Time since treatment	-	-	−0.006	−0.063	−0.013	−0.136
Type of treatment	-	-	−0.085	−0.854	−0.065	−0.674
Pain	-	-	−0.072	−0.676	−0.029	−0.273
Fatigue	-	-	0.046	0.436	0.044	0.416
Hardiness	-	-	-	-	0.134	0.898
Coping	-	-	-	-	−0.164	−1.236
Adaptability	-	-	-	-	0.267	2.092 *
Meaningfulness	-	-	-	-	−0.371	−2.648 *
Optimism	-	-	-	-	0.138	1.331
Regulation of emotion and cognition	-	-	-	-	0.248	2.328 *
Self-efficacy	-	-	-	-	0.104	0.859

* $p < 0.05$.

Table 7. Mediator effect of sociodemographic, clinical characteristics, and resilience to the expression of perceived instrumental support.

	Step 1 $F = 1.83$, $p = 0.090$, $R^2 = 0.05$		Step 2 $F = 1.61, p = 0.100$, $R^2 = 0.07, \Delta R^2 = 0.02$, $p = 0.260$		Step 3 $F = 2.29, p = 0.010$, $R^2 = 0.20, \Delta R^2 = 0.13$, $p = 0.006$	
	β	t	β	t	β	t
Age	−0.084	−0.833	−0.073	−0.699	−0.118	−1.197
Education	−0.214	−1.922	−0.202	−1.811	−0.238	−2.275 *
Professional activity	0.235	2.166	0.181	1.601	0.067	0.616
Residence	−0.096	−0.860	−0.109	−0.938	−0.048	−0.431
Self-reported financial standing	0.257	2.356	0.228	2.094	0.196	1.867
Partner	0.128	1.120	0.112	0.970	0.062	0.561
Stress	-	-	0.015	0.137	0.069	0.674
Time since treatment	-	-	0.013	0.119	0.049	0.475
Type of treatment	-	-	0.078	0.752	−0.035	−0.348
Pain	-	-	−0.088	−0.792	0.047	0.410
Fatigue	-	-	−0.170	−1.540	−0.091	−0.831
Hardiness	-	-	-	-	0.105	0.672
Coping	-	-	-	-	0.132	0.925
Adaptability	-	-	-	-	0.240	1.762
Meaningfulness	-	-	-	-	−0.012	−0.080
Optimism	-	-	-	-	−0.053	−0.489
Regulation of emotion and cognition	-	-	-	-	−0.002	−0.015
Self-efficacy	-	-	-	-	0.146	1.168

* $p < 0.05$.

Table 8. Mediator effect of sociodemographic, clinical characteristics, and resilience to the expression of actual received emotional social support.

	Step 1 $F = 0.90$, $p = 0.051$, $R^2 = 0.06$		Step 2 $F = 1.19, p = 0.300$, $R^2 = 0.15, \Delta R^2 = 0.09$, $p = 0.192$		Step 3 $F = 1.97, p = 0.020$, $R^2 = 0.32, \Delta R^2 = 0.17$, $p = 0.006$	
	β	t	β	t	β	t
Age	−0.021	−0.193	0.007	0.066	−0.027	−0.265
Education	−0.084	−0.718	−0.033	−0.277	−0.070	−0.632
Professional activity	0.177	1.558	0.182	1.542	0.078	0.674
Residence	−0.189	−1.589	−0.235	−1.902	−0.199	−1.662
Self-reported financial standing	0.207	1.788	0.178	1.536	0.138	1.249
Partner	0.010	0.088	0.006	0.055	−0.047	−0.890
Stress	-	-	−0.111	−0.995	−0.200	−0.447
Time since treatment	-	-	−0.247	−2.265	−0.061	−1.901
Type of treatment	-	-	0.007	0.062	−0.589	−0.589
Pain	-	-	−0.041	−0.352	−0.023	−0.195
Fatigue	-	-	−0.141	−1.223	−0.014	−0.119
Hardiness	-	-	-	-	0.410	2.483
Coping	-	-	-	-	−0.018	−0.127
Adaptability	-	-	-	-	0.189	1.363
Meaningfulness	-	-	-	-	−0.060	−0.388
Optimism	-	-	-	-	0.053	0.465
Regulation of emotion and cognition	-	-	-	-	−0.142	−1.236
Self-efficacy	-	-	-	-	0.001	0.006

4. Discussion

Social support can be viewed as an interactive construct, an interpersonal transaction that occurs between those who need help and those who provide support [29].

The importance of social support in improving positive treatment outcomes for people with chronic diseases and conditions has been confirmed in previous research [11,16,19,23]. Studies have shown that cancer patients who have higher levels of social support have a better quality of life and lower mortality rates [30,31]. Social support has been identified as one of the key factors in the daily lives of cancer patients [32]. Therefore, one of the aims of our study was to determine the level of social support in patients with breast cancer. The results of our research indicate a relatively high level of received social support [3.51 ± 0.63], which is in accordance with the results of previous studies [18,33]. It is common knowledge that many patients with cancer or other chronic diseases resort to their own network of social support and use different methods of self-management when faced with stressful situations. The reason for this might be the traditional family structure, which is still commonly present in Serbia. Dedication of family members and relatives to each other and good relationships with neighbors, particularly in difficult circumstances, such as disease, can be a significant factor, potentially impacting the results of this study. A higher level of social support after a breast cancer diagnosis can be valuable for the survival of these women because it improves their coping skills and increases the availability of cancer-related information [34]. The effects of social support suggest that it mainly operates as a stress alleviation model, with the greatest and most reliable benefits of support under conditions of psychological stress when support is most needed [12]. Observing the sociodemographic and clinical data of patients can provide relevant information on risk and protective factors that influence the adjustment to cancer diagnosis [35]. The results of our study suggest that age and a lower level of education contribute to increasing the need for social support. In contrast, the level of social support remains the same regardless of the partnership relationship, socioeconomic status, employment, and whether someone lives in urban or rural areas. Older cancer patients are faced with multiple challenges that include multiple losses, such as loss of strength to accomplish some of their routine activities at home, practical tasks, or social contacts [34]. Even when they receive support, these older women still suffer because of the loss of functional independence [36–38]. Unlike our results, a study conducted in Poland found that the education level did not influence the need for support among the participants [39], whereas living in urban areas was a positive and independent predictor of social support among survivors in China [40]. Our study also showed a higher score in the domain of protective buffering support among the employed participants. They proved to be protective of their environment regarding the information about the disease and diagnosis. These findings suggest that the social roles that confirm self-worth within the family, friends, or at work are extremely important for female social support experience [41,42]. The results of previous studies indicate that in the breast cancer patient population, work increases self-worth, quality of life, sense of purpose, and social integration [41]. In addition, such findings may indicate the presence of stigma related to the diagnosis and breast cancer treatment. It is necessary to conduct further research to provide closer insight into the matter. Among clinical variables, significant predictors of social support were the elapsed time since the treatment, the type of treatment, pain, fatigue, and stress. For some cancer patients, the amount of support can change over time, which indicates that the level and the type of support should be monitored. Namely, if the period of time since the treatment is short, there is a higher need for support [43]. Our study confirmed that the longer the treatment lasted, the less support they felt. Regarding different therapeutic treatment methods, experiencing systemic therapy is the factor that mostly impacted the increased level of seeking support and the higher level of satisfaction with the support. These findings are in accordance with previous studies [42]. Fatigue, pain, and stress can dramatically affect the quality of life of breast cancer patients, making them too exhausted to participate in regular activities and social events. In our study, participants who were without pain, fatigue, and stress reported significantly higher levels of social support. These results support earlier findings that found that women who reported higher levels of social support also reported lower levels of fatigue and pain [44,45]. Women with breast cancer can report varying levels of pain interference independent of pain intensity. Psychosocial factors, such as social support, may impact patients' levels of pain interference. One of the significant psychosocial factors connected to negative emotional reactions of breast cancer patients is their psychological resilience. It is not about one personal characteristic but the result of an interaction between multiple personal characteristics and environmental factors [12]. Recent studies emphasize that psychological resilience as a personal factor and social support as an environmental factor function as a buffer against stress and increase the quality of life by reducing emotional stress among cancer patients [46,47]. Studies have found that resilience can strongly predict the patients' fatigue from treatment, and well-developed resilience can help patients reduce treatment-induced functional impairment and shorten recovery time [48,49]. Coping style in oncology has been proven as one of the central factors in modulating the different individual psychological reactions towards the disease, the quality of life after receiving a cancer diagnosis, and the response and adjustment to treatment. The results of the correlation analysis of resilience and social support show a strong positive relationship. Namely, the more resilient female participants were, the higher the level of social support they received. The obtained results completely correspond to previously published studies [50]. Highly resilient cancer patients can depend less on psychosocial support in stress management when compared to those with lower resilience [51]. It is clear that social support improves general well-being, minimizes the risk of psychological stress, and represents a key factor in increasing the sense of hope among patients who have been diagnosed with cancer [52]. However, in our study, resilience did not function as a mediator in patients' total social support and sociodemographic and clinical characteristics. Its potential mediating role was only found in the domain of seeking support and actually receiving emotional social support.

5. Conclusions

The obtained results serve as a fundamental basis for the development of a support system for breast cancer patients during and after treatment. Nurses should pay more attention to the resilience status and level of social support, as well as the coping style demonstrated by breast cancer patients. Methods and models of social support need to be adjusted to patients according to age and level of education. Identifying risk factors and inadequate coping mechanisms and creating social support programs targeting patients and their families so they can express their thoughts and feelings are vital. Further research is needed to identify factors that contribute to social support for breast cancer patients.

Limitations of This Study

Our research faced several limitations. To begin with, it was a cross-sectional study, whereas a longitudinal approach would be more suitable for monitoring the changes in perceptions and needs for social support over time. Another limitation is related to the need to expand the group of participants, which could be achieved by introducing a comparative analysis with male breast cancer patients. Ultimately, we found a significant correlation between resilience and social support, but more research is needed to fully understand this relationship.

Author Contributions: Conceptualization, S.D.T., G.M. and A.Š.; Methodology, S.D.T., G.M., A.Š., E.M. and S.T.; Software, A.Š.; Validation, E.M.; Formal analysis, S.D.T., S.T. and G.M.; Investigation, S.D.T., G.M., A.Š., E.M. and S.T.; Resources, S.D.T., E.M. and S.T.; Data curation, G.M. and A.Š.; Writing—original draft, A.Š., S.D.T. and S.T.; Writing—review and editing, S.D.T., G.M., A.Š., E.M. and S.T.; Visualization, E.M.; Supervision, S.D.T., G.M. and E.M.; Project administration, S.D.T., G.M., A.Š., E.M. and S.T. All authors have read and agreed to the published version of the manuscript.

Funding: This research received no external funding.

Institutional Review Board Statement: This study was approved by the Ethics Committee of the Faculty of Medicine in Novi Sad (01-39/34/1/2023) and the Ethics Committee of the "Dr. Radivoj Simonović" General Hospital in Sombor (23-3108/2023).

Informed Consent Statement: Informed consent was obtained from all subjects involved in this study.

Data Availability Statement: The data are available from the authors on personal request.

Conflicts of Interest: The authors declare no conflict of interest.

References

1. Siegel, R.L.; Miller, K.D.; Fuchs, H.E.; Jemal, A. Cancer statistics, 2021. *CA Cancer J. Clin.* **2021**, *71*, 7–33. [CrossRef] [PubMed]
2. Sung, H.; Ferlay, J.; Siegel, R.L.; Laversanne, M.; Soerjomataram, I.; Jemal, A.; Bray, F. Global cancer statistics 2020: GLOBOCAN estimates of incidence and mortality worldwide for 36 cancers in 185 countries. *CA Cancer J. Clin.* **2021**, *71*, 209–249. [CrossRef] [PubMed]
3. Zhang, H.; Xiao, L.; Ren, G. Experiences of social support among Chinese women with breast cancer: A qualitative analysis using a framework approach. *Med. Sci. Monit.* **2018**, *24*, 574–581. [CrossRef] [PubMed]
4. Park, J.H.; Chun, M.; Jung, Y.S.; Bae, S.H. Predictors of psychological distress trajectories in the first year after a breast cancer diagnosis. *Asian Nurs. Res.* **2017**, *11*, 268–275. [CrossRef] [PubMed]
5. Spatuzzi, R.; Vespa, A.; Lorenzi, P.; Miccinesi, G.; Ricciuti, M.; Cifarelli, W.; Susi, M.; Fabrizio, T.; Ferrari, M.G.; Ottaviani, M.; et al. Evaluation of social support, quality of life, and body image in women with breast cancer. *Breast Care* **2016**, *11*, 28–32. [CrossRef] [PubMed]
6. Mokhatri-Hesari, P.; Montazeri, A. Health-related quality of life in breast cancer patients: Review of reviews from 2008 to 2018. *Health Qual. Life Outcomes* **2020**, *18*, 338. [CrossRef]
7. Hashemi, S.M.; Balouchi, A.; Al-Mawali, A.; Rafiemanesh, H.; Rezaie-Keikhaie, K.; Bouya, S.; Dehghan, B.; Farahani, M.A. Health-related quality of life of breast cancer patients in the eastern Mediterranean region: A systematic review and meta-analysis. *Breast Cancer Res. Treat.* **2019**, *174*, 585–596. [CrossRef]
8. El Haidari, R.; Abbas, L.A.; Nerich, V.; Anota, A. Factors associated with health-related quality of life in women with breast cancer in the Middle East: A systematic review. *Cancers* **2020**, *12*, 696. [CrossRef]
9. Sousa, H.; Castro, S.; Abreu, J.; Pereira, M.G. A systematic review of factors affecting quality of life after postmastectomy breast reconstruction in women with breast cancer. *Psychooncology* **2019**, *28*, 2107–2118. [CrossRef]
10. Çelik, G.K.; Çakır, H.; Kut, E. Mediating Role of Social Support in Resilience and Quality of Life in Patients with Breast Cancer: Structural Equation Model Analysis. *Asia Pac. J. Oncol. Nurs.* **2020**, *8*, 86–93. [CrossRef]
11. Abdollahi, A.; Alsaikhan, F.; Nikolenko, D.A.; Al-Gazally, M.E.; Mahmudiono, T.; Allen, K.A.; Abdullaev, B. Self-care behaviors mediates the relationship between resilience and quality of life in breast cancer patients. *BMC Psychiatry* **2022**, *22*, 825. [CrossRef] [PubMed]
12. Cohen, S.; Gottlieb, B.H.; Underwood, L.G. Social relationships and health: Challenges for measurement and intervention. *Adv. Mind Body Med.* **2001**, *17*, 129–141. [CrossRef] [PubMed]
13. Schwarzer, R.; Leppin, A. Social support and health: A theoretical and empirical overview. *J. Soc. Pers. Relat.* **1991**, *8*, 99–127. [CrossRef]
14. Cohen, S.; Wills, T.A. Stress, social support, and the buffering hypothesis. *Psychol. Bull.* **1985**, *98*, 310–357. [CrossRef] [PubMed]
15. National Cancer Institute. NCI Dictionary of Cancer Terms. Available online: www.cancer.gov/publications/dictionaries/cancer-terms/def/social-support (accessed on 26 October 2023).
16. Barrera, M. Distinctions between social support concepts, measures, and models. *Am. J. Comm. Psychol.* **1986**, *14*, 413–445. [CrossRef]
17. Helgeson, V.S.; Cohen, S. Social support and adjustment to cancer: Reconciling descriptive, correlational, and intervention research. *Health Psychol.* **1996**, *15*, 135–148. [CrossRef] [PubMed]
18. Schulz, U.; Schwarzer, R. Soziale Unterstützung bei der Krankheitsbewältigung: Die Berliner Social Support Skalen (BSSS) [Social support in coping with illness: The Berlin Social Support Scales (BSSS)]. *Diagnostica* **2003**, *49*, 73–82. [CrossRef]
19. Almuhtaseb, M.I.A.; Alby, F.; Zuccermaglio, C.; Fatigante, M. Social support for breast cancer patients in the occupied Palestinian territory. *PLoS ONE* **2021**, *16*, e0252608. [CrossRef]
20. Ozdemir, D.; Arslan, F.T. An investigation of the relationship between social support and coping with stress in women with breast cancer. *Psychooncology* **2018**, *27*, 2214–2219. [CrossRef]
21. Padilla-Ruiz, M.; Ruiz-Román, C.; Pérez-Ruiz, E.; Rueda, A.; Redondo, M.; Rivas-Ruiz, F. Clinical and sociodemographic factors that may influence the resilience of women surviving breast cancer: Cross-sectional study. *Support. Care Cancer* **2019**, *27*, 1279–1286. [CrossRef]
22. Naik, H.; Leung, B.; Laskin, J.; McDonald, M.; Srikanthan, A.; Wu, J.; Bates, A.; Ho, C. Emotional distress and psychosocial needs in patients with breast cancer in British Columbia: Younger versus older adults. *Breast Cancer Res. Treat.* **2020**, *179*, 471–477. [CrossRef] [PubMed]

23. Champion, V.L.; Wagner, L.I.; Monahan, P.O.; Daggy, J.; Smith, L.; Cohee, A.; Ziner, K.W.; Haase, J.E.; Miller, K.D.; Pradhan, K.; et al. Compariosn of younger and older breast cancer survivors and age-matched controls on specific overall quality of life domains. *Cancer* **2014**, *120*, 2237–2246. [CrossRef]
24. Bonanno, G.A.; Westphal, M.; Mancini, A.D. Resilience to loss and potential trauma. *Annu. Rev. Clin. Psychol.* **2011**, *7*, 511–535. [CrossRef] [PubMed]
25. Eicher, M.; Matzka, M.; Dubey, C.; White, K. Resilience in adult cancer care: An integrative literature review. *Oncol. Nurs. Forum.* **2015**, *42*, E3–E16. [CrossRef] [PubMed]
26. Simasundaram, R.O.; Devamani, K.A. A Comparative Study on Resilience, Perceived Social Support and Hopelessness Among Cancer Patients Treated with Curative and Palliative Care. *Indian. J. Palliat. Care* **2016**, *2*, 135–140. [CrossRef] [PubMed]
27. Schwartz, A.L.; Meek, P.M.; Nail, L.M.; Fargo, J.; Lundquist, M.; Donofrio, M.; Grainger, M.; Throckmorton, T.; Mateo, M. Measurement of fatigue. determining minimally important clinical differences. *J. Clin. Epidemiol.* **2002**, *55*, 239–244. [CrossRef] [PubMed]
28. Wills, T.A.; Shinar, O. Measuring perceived and received social support. In *Social Support Measurement and Intervention: A Guide for Health and Social Scientists*; Cohen, S., Underwood, L.G., Gottlieb, B.H., Eds.; Oxford University Press: Oxford, UK, 2020; pp. 86–135. [CrossRef]
29. Ruiz-Rodríguez, I.; Hombrados-Mendieta, I.; Melguizo-Garín, A.; Martos-Méndez, M.J. The Importance of Social Support, Optimism and Resilience on the Quality of Life of Cancer Patients. *Front. Psychol.* **2022**, *13*, 833176. [CrossRef]
30. Corovic, S.; Vucic, V.; Mihaljevic, O.; Djordjevic, J.; Colovic, S.; Radovanovic, S.; Radevic, S.; Vukomanovic, I.S.; Janicijevic, K.; Sekulic, M.; et al. Social support score in patients with malignant diseases-with sociodemographic and medical characteristics. *Front. Psychol.* **2023**, *14*, 1160020. [CrossRef]
31. Usta, Y.Y. Importance of social support in cancer patients. *Asian Pac. J. Cancer Prev.* **2012**, *13*, 3569–3572. [CrossRef]
32. Lu, D.; Andersson, T.M.; Fall, K.; Hultman, C.M.; Czene, K.; Valdimarsdóttir, U.; Fang, F. Clinical Diagnosis of Mental Disorders Immediately Before and After Cancer Diagnosis: A Nationwide Matched Cohort Study in Sweden. *JAMA Oncol.* **2016**, *2*, 1188–1196. [CrossRef]
33. DiMillo, J.; Hall, N.C.; Ezer, H.; Schwarzer, R.; Körner, A. The Berlin Social Support Scales: Validation of the Received Support Scale in a Canadian sample of patients affected by melanoma. *J. Health Psychol.* **2019**, *24*, 1785–1795. [CrossRef] [PubMed]
34. Zhu, J.; Sjölander, A.; Fall, K.; Valdimarsdottir, U.; Fang, F. Mental disorders around cancer diagnosis and increased hospital admission rate—A nationwide cohort study of Swedish cancer patients. *BMC Cancer* **2018**, *18*, 322. [CrossRef] [PubMed]
35. Faraci, P.; Bottaro, R. A Cross-Sectional Study Examining the Relationship Between Socio-Demographics and Coping Styles in a Group of Cancer Patients. *Clin. Neuropsychiatry* **2021**, *18*, 3–12. [CrossRef] [PubMed]
36. Posma, E.R.; van Weert, J.C.; Jansen, J.; Bensing, J.M. Older cancer patients' information and support needs surrounding treatment: An evaluation through the eyes of patients, relatives and professionals. *BMC Nurs.* **2009**, *8*, 1. [CrossRef] [PubMed]
37. Yancik, R.; Wesley, M.N.; Ries, L.A.; Havlik, R.J.; Edwards, B.K.; Yates, J.W. Effect of age and comorbidity in postmenopausal breast cancer patients aged 55 years and older. *JAMA* **2001**, *285*, 885–892. [CrossRef] [PubMed]
38. Wyatt, G.; Beckrow, K.C.; Gardiner, J.; Pathak, D. Predictors of postsurgical subacute emotional and physical well-being among women with breast cancer. *Cancer Nurs.* **2008**, *31*, E28–E39. [CrossRef]
39. Pasek, M.; Suchocka, L.; Gąsior, K. Model of Social Support for Patients Treated for Cancer. *Cancers* **2021**, *13*, 4786. [CrossRef]
40. Zhou, K.; Ning, F.; Wang, W.; Li, X. The mediator role of resilience between psychological predictors and health-related quality of life in breast cancer survivors: A cross-sectional study. *BMC Cancer* **2022**, *22*, 57. [CrossRef]
41. Costa-Requena, G.; Ballester Arnal, R.; Gil, F. Perceived social support in Spanish cancer outpatients with psychiatric disorder. *Stress. Health* **2013**, *29*, 421–426. [CrossRef]
42. Matchim, Y.; Armer, J.M.; Stewart, B.R. Mindfulness-based stress reduction among breast cancer survivors: A literature review and discussion. *Oncol. Nurs. Forum.* **2011**, *38*, E61–E71. [CrossRef]
43. Yılmaz, S.D.; Bal, M.D.; Beji, N.K.; Arvas, M. Ways of coping with stress and perceived social support in gynecologic cancer patients. *Cancer Nurs.* **2015**, *38*, E57–E62. [CrossRef] [PubMed]
44. Bloom, J.R.; Stewart, S.L.; Johnston, M.; Banks, P.; Fobair, P. Sources of social Support and the physical and mental well-being of young women with breast cancer. *Soc. Sci. Med.* **2001**, *53*, 1513–1524. [CrossRef] [PubMed]
45. Fisher, H.M.; Winger, J.G.; Miller, S.N.; Wright, A.N.; Plumb Vilardaga, J.C.; Majestic, C.; Kelleher, S.A.; Somers, T.J. Relationship between social support, physical symptoms, and depression in women with breast cancer and pain. *Support. Care Cancer* **2021**, *29*, 5513–5521. [CrossRef] [PubMed]
46. Zhang, H.; Zhao, Q.; Cao, P.; Ren, G. Resilience and Quality of Life: Exploring the Mediator Role of Social Support in Patients with Breast Cancer. *Med. Sci. Monit.* **2017**, *23*, 5969–5979. [CrossRef] [PubMed]
47. Min, J.A.; Yoon, S.; Lee, C.U.; Chae, J.H.; Lee, C.; Song, K.Y.; Kim, T.S. Psychological resilience contributes to low emotional distress in cancer patients. *Support. Care Cancer* **2013**, *21*, 2469–2476. [CrossRef] [PubMed]
48. Wenzel, L.B.; Donnelly, J.P.; Fowler, J.M.; Habbal, R.; Taylor, T.H.; Aziz, N.; Cella, D. Resilience, reflection, and residual stress in ovarian cancer survivorship: A gynecologic oncology group study. *Psychooncology* **2002**, *11*, 142–153. [CrossRef]
49. Strauss, B.; Brix, C.; Fischer, S.; Leppert, K.; Füller, J.; Roehrig, B.; Schleussner, C.; Wendt, T.G. The influence of resilience on fatigue in cancer patients undergoing radiation therapy (RT). *J. Cancer Res. Clin. Oncol.* **2007**, *133*, 511–518. [CrossRef]

50. Yoo, G.J.; Levine, E.G.; Aviv, C.; Ewing, C.; Au, A. Older women, breast cancer, and social support. *Support. Care Cancer* **2010**, *18*, 1521–1530. [CrossRef]
51. Koopman, C.; Angell, K.; Turner-Cobb, J.M.; Kreshka, M.A.; Donnelly, P.; McCoy, R.; Turkseven, A.; Graddy, K.; Giese-Davis, J.; Spiegel, D. Distress, coping, and social support among rural women recently diagnosed with primary breast cancer. *Breast J.* **2001**, *7*, 25–33. [CrossRef]
52. Smith, S.K.; Herndon, J.E.; Lyerly, H.K.; Coan, A.; Wheeler, J.L.; Staley, T.; Abernethy, A.P. Correlates of quality of life-related outcomes in breast cancer patients participating in the Pathfinders pilot study. *Psychooncology* **2011**, *20*, 559–564. [CrossRef]

Disclaimer/Publisher's Note: The statements, opinions and data contained in all publications are solely those of the individual author(s) and contributor(s) and not of MDPI and/or the editor(s). MDPI and/or the editor(s) disclaim responsibility for any injury to people or property resulting from any ideas, methods, instructions or products referred to in the content.

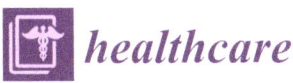

Article

Effects of Post Traumatic Growth on Successful Aging in Breast Cancer Survivors in South Korea: The Mediating Effect of Resilience and Intolerance of Uncertainty

Su Jeong Yi [1], Ku Sang Kim [2], Seunghee Lee [1,*] and Hyunjung Lee [3,*]

1. College of Nursing, Dankook University, Cheonan 31116, Republic of Korea; 12181056@dankook.ac.kr
2. Department of Breast Surgery, Kosin University Gospel Hospital, Busan 49267, Republic of Korea; ideakims@gmail.com
3. College of Nursing, Chungnam National University, Daejeon 35015, Republic of Korea
* Correspondence: 12191010@dankook.ac.kr (S.L.); leehj22@cnu.ac.kr (H.L.)

Abstract: This study aimed to identify post-traumatic growth and successful aging and the mediating effects of resilience and intolerance of uncertainty in breast cancer survivors. This study employed a descriptive survey approach. Data were collected from 143 breast cancer survivors between 27 January and 10 December 2021, at a cancer center in Gyeongsangnam-do, South Korea. SPSS/WIN 25.0 and PROCESS Macro version 3.5 were used for data analysis. Descriptive statistics were analyzed with SPSS. PROCESS was used to conduct a mediation analysis and the significance of the mediating effect was evaluated using 95% confidence intervals. Successful aging was significantly associated with post-traumatic growth, resilience, and the intolerance of uncertainty. The impact of post-traumatic growth on successful aging was mediated by resilience in breast cancer survivors. Resilience should be considered when developing nursing interventions to enhance post-traumatic growth and promote successful aging in breast cancer survivors.

Keywords: breast cancer; post traumatic growth; resilience; intolerance of uncertainty; nursing intervention

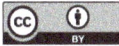

Citation: Yi, S.J.; Kim, K.S.; Lee, S.; Lee, H. Effects of Post Traumatic Growth on Successful Aging in Breast Cancer Survivors in South Korea: The Mediating Effect of Resilience and Intolerance of Uncertainty. *Healthcare* **2023**, *11*, 2843. https://doi.org/10.3390/healthcare11212843

Academic Editor: Qiuping Li

Received: 6 September 2023
Revised: 23 October 2023
Accepted: 26 October 2023
Published: 28 October 2023

Copyright: © 2023 by the authors. Licensee MDPI, Basel, Switzerland. This article is an open access article distributed under the terms and conditions of the Creative Commons Attribution (CC BY) license (https://creativecommons.org/licenses/by/4.0/).

1. Introduction

The incidence of patients with breast cancer in South Korea increased at an average annual rate of 4.3% from 2007 to 2019. Breast cancer has a high survival rate, with a five-year relative survival rate of 93.6% after a diagnosis [1]. The average age of patients with breast cancer at diagnosis is 52.5 (±8.23) years; the highest incidence occurs in individuals in their 40 s, with a growing number of cases reported in those who are in their 50 s and beyond [2].

The increasing incidence of breast cancer and the extended average survival time after diagnosis means that there will be a growing number of breast cancer survivors who will live longer. With an the increase in the breast cancer survival rate, many patients are becoming more concerned about their long-term health, including the quality of life and successful aging after cancer. Therefore, there is a need for attention to successful aging in later life among cancer survivors who have returned to their daily lives [3]. Successful aging is an individual's sense of having adapted to the physiological and functional changes associated with the passage of time, while also finding meaning or purpose in life [4]. Successful aging is a broad, complex concept that encompasses attributes of both physical and psychological health [5] and means having a low risk of disease and disability, maintaining high levels of physical and mental functioning, and actively participating in life [6]. Patients with breast cancer undergo aggressive treatment-including chemotherapy-depending on the stage of the cancer, even after surgery, owing to the risk of cancer metastasis and recurrence. After treatment ends, they could have many negative experiences, such as treatment side effects, complications, and changes in femininity [7]. As breast cancer survivors age, they simultaneously experience the functional and physiological challenges associated with the normal aging process, as well as the various challenges associated with treatment. Therefore, their aging process is believed to require more active management and care. Focusing on the strategies and processes of successful aging, that is, coping with life after treatment and providing appropriate interventions, is vital [8]. Flood's theory [4] of successful aging, considers it an adaptation of functional performance, intrapsychic factors and spirituality; intrapsychic factors refer to an individual's character that can enhance or impair their ability to adapt to change and solve problems. Therefore, successful aging requires an exploration of the individual's character. Consequently, this study seeks to provide an integrated understanding of the psychological mechanisms that influence successful aging.

Post-traumatic growth is associated with adaptation and successful aging in patients with cancer [8]. Further, in a study of middle-aged women, post-traumatic growth was a positive predictor of successful aging. Post-traumatic growth is defined as psychological well-being resulting from the positive adjustment to trauma [9], and a previous study [10] has shown that psychological well-being is significantly and positively related to successful aging. Therefore, it is expected that there is a significant relationship between post-traumatic growth and successful aging. Post-traumatic growth is the positive change in perceptions of self, others, and life after a traumatic event and includes changes in self-perception, interpersonal relationships, and life stance [11]. As they enter remission after the end of medical treatment, many breast cancer survivors experience physical symptoms such as lymphedema, pain, and fatigue, as well as mental distress such as depression and fear of recurrence [12]. However, in addition to these negative aspects, breast cancer survivors experience positive changes such as an increased appreciation for life, setting life goals, and discovering their strengths [13,14]. These changes can be referred to as post-traumatic growth; from a human developmental perspective, effective strategies to promote and sustain post-traumatic growth are needed for successful transition and adaptation to older age as a breast cancer survivor [13]. This is because post-traumatic growth in patients with cancer is a major factor in improving their coping skills, enabling them to actively face challenges, and ultimately elevating their level of successful aging in the future. If post-traumatic growth influences successful aging, how is the relationship between the two variables established? If we introduce a mediator in the relationship between these independent and dependent variables, we can understand the "how" in the relationship between the two variables [15]. By utilizing a mediation model, we can examine the internal psychological resources an individual possesses to foster successful aging and understand its mechanism.

We selected resilience as the first parameter. A key concept that could reduce negative outcomes through positive coping is resilience in breast cancer survivors [16]. Resilience is defined as the ability to return to an original state after being modified by an external force [16]. It refers to the ability to psychologically overcome adversity, leading to positive outcomes or reducing negative outcomes [17]. Post-traumatic growth and resilience are correlated [18,19]. An important factor in successful aging, despite the various changes throughout the life cycle, is individuals' resilience [20]. Jeste et al. [21] reported that higher levels of resilience are associated with higher successful aging scores in the elderly; thus, it is worthwhile to explore the mediating effect of resilience on the relationship between post-traumatic growth and successful aging in breast cancer survivors. In addition, previous studies have indicated that there is either a negative correlation between resilience and the intolerance of uncertainty [22], or resilience on intolerance of uncertainty [23]. This suggests a need for further exploration of their relationship.

The study also highlighted intolerance of uncertainty as another variable. Since cancer progression and prognosis cannot be predicted with certainty, cancer survivors must endure uncertainty, both in general and in specific aspects related to the disease [24]. Particularly for breast cancer, in which survival rates are high, intolerance of uncertainty can lead to negative reactions across cognitive, emotional, and behavioral domains to stimuli or situations that arise in everyday life [25]. People with intolerance of uncertainty perceive and respond negatively to uncertain information and situations, regardless of probability or outcome [26], and they demonstrate increased psychological distress when faced with ambiguous symptoms [27]. Previous studies revealed that intolerance of uncertainty about disease prognosis was also associated with depressive symptoms [28,29], health anxiety, and anxiety sensitivity in female patients with breast cancer [30]. However, most previous research has focused on understanding the association between disease-related uncertainty and psychological outcomes [28–30]. In addition, the scant literature has explored the impact of intolerance of uncertainty as a factor related to cognitive, emotional, and behavioral responses to post-traumatic growth and successful aging in breast cancer survivors.

Antonovsky's [31,32] Generalized Resistance Resource (GRRs) theory primarily addresses how individuals maintain health and adapt when confronted with stress or challenges. Antonovsky [31,32] suggested that GRRs are resources or abilities that assist individuals in coping with negative situations such as stress or illness. Post-traumatic growth can be viewed as an indicator of the GRRs that breast cancer survivors acquire after experiencing trauma. Resilience can be considered a GRR, and intolerance of uncertainty can be considered an indicator of a lack of or insufficient GRRs. Post-traumatic growth will enhance resilience and reduce intolerance of uncertainty. This enhanced resilience and reduced intolerance of uncertainty will promote successful aging.

In the existing research, there is a dearth of studies examining the relationship between post-traumatic growth and successful aging among breast cancer survivors, especially the mediating effect of intolerance of uncertainty and resilience. To address this research gap, this study explores the relationship between post-traumatic growth and successful aging among breast cancer survivors from a new perspective and reveals the important role of intolerance of uncertainty and resilience. The specific aims were (a) to examine correlations among variables, including post-traumatic growth, successful aging, intolerance of uncertainty, and resilience; and (b) to examine the serial multiple mediation of resilience, and intolerance of uncertainty between post-traumatic growth and successful aging. The serial multiple mediator model has the advantage of providing a more comprehensive understanding of psychological mechanisms by examining the previously individually studied variables within a model that includes two mediating variables [15]. It is expected that this will provide insights into the process of improving quality of life and successful aging among breast cancer survivors.

2. Materials and Methods

2.1. Study Design

This was a descriptive correlational study.

2.2. Participants

Participants were adult women living in the Busan and Gyeongnam regions who had been diagnosed with breast cancer. Specific inclusion criteria were as follows: over-middle-aged women, aged 40 years or older, who understood the study purpose and agreed to participate; those who were diagnosed with breast cancer and underwent mastectomy or partial mastectomy; and those who completed adjuvant treatments such as chemotherapy (excluding hormone therapy) and radiation therapy, or no longer required adjuvant treatment after surgery.

The number of participants was calculated using G*Power 3.1.9.4. For a hierarchical regression analysis, a minimum sample size of 129 was calculated with a significance level (α) of 0.05, effect size (f^2) of 0.15, power ($1 - \beta$) of 0.80, and 10 predictors (general characteristics_age, religious state, and employment status; disease-related characteristics_treatment period, activity ability and symptomatic state; post-traumatic growth, successful aging, intolerance of uncertainty, and resilience) based on previous research [33,34]. One hundred and fifty people were surveyed, considering a 10% dropout rate. A total of 143 copies of the survey were analyzed, excluding 7 copies with insufficient responses.

2.3. Measures

2.3.1. Post-Traumatic Growth

Post-traumatic growth was measured using the Korean Version of the Post-traumatic Growth Inventory developed by Tedeschi and Calhoun [11], which was modified by Song Seung-hoon et al. [35]. This scale measured the extent to which one agrees with positive changes after a traumatic experience on a six-point scale ranging from 0 to 5 points, with higher scores indicating more positive changes after a traumatic experience. At the time of scale development, Cronbach's $\alpha = 0.90$. In this study, Cronbach's $\alpha = 0.93$, indicating excellent internal consistency.

2.3.2. Successful Aging

Successful aging was measured using the Successful Aging Inventory developed by Troutman et al. [36], which was modified and supplemented by Jang Hyung-sook [37]. A five-point scale from 0 to 4 points was developed, with higher scores indicating higher levels of successful aging. At the time of scale development, Cronbach's $\alpha = 0.86$. In the study of Jang Hyung-sook [37], Cronbach's $\alpha = 0.93$. In this study, Cronbach's $\alpha = 0.93$, indicating excellent internal consistency.

2.3.3. Intolerance of Uncertainty

Intolerance of uncertainty was measured using the Intolerance of Uncertainty Scale by Freeston et al. [24], which was adapted into Korean by Choi Hye-kyung [38]. The scale consists of 27 items scored on a four-point Likert scale, with higher scores indicating higher levels of intolerance of uncertainty. At the time of scale development, Cronbach's $\alpha = 0.91$. In this study, Cronbach's $\alpha = 0.95$, indicating excellent internal consistency.

2.3.4. Resilience

Resilience was measured using the Connor–Davidson Resilience Scale 2, developed by Vaushnavi, Connor, and Davidson [39], after obtaining the Korean version from the developer with permission to use the scale. The scale consisted of two items scored on a five-point scale (0–4 points), with higher scores indicating higher levels of resilience. At the time of scale development, Cronbach's $\alpha = 0.89$. In this study, Cronbach's $\alpha = 0.78$, indicating acceptable internal consistency.

2.4. Data Collection

Data were collected from 21 January to 10 December 2021, after obtaining the approval of the Institutional Review Board of Kosin University Gospel Hospital (no: 2020-12-020). With the hospital's permission, patients who met the inclusion criteria were referred by their physicians; the first and third authors personally explained the study purpose and sought patients' consent to participate before or after the start of their medical care. Those who expressed their willingness to participate were given a consent form and asked to complete a questionnaire. The informed consent form specified the purpose, procedures, and methods, the method of participation and the capacity to withdraw at any time, and the protection of personal information. On average, it took 15 to 20 min to complete the questionnaire; if it was difficult for the participant to complete the questionnaire by themselves, the authors read the questionnaire to them and completed it for them. Completed questionnaires were sealed in a paper envelope to protect privacy and collected by the authors. In return for completing the survey, a gift coupon of 10,000 won (approximately 10 US dollars) was given to participants.

2.5. Data Analysis

Data were analyzed using SPSS 25.0 (IBM, Armonk, NY, USA) and PROCESS Macro version 3.5. General and disease-related characteristics, post-traumatic growth, successful aging, resilience, and intolerance of uncertainty were measured using descriptive statistics. Differences in post-traumatic growth, successful aging, resilience, and intolerance of uncertainty according to general characteristics were analyzed with *t*-tests and analyses of variance, with Scheffé's post hoc tests. Correlations between post-traumatic growth, successful aging, resilience, and intolerance of uncertainty were analyzed using Pearson's correlation tests. To testing the serial multiple mediation analysis, Process Macro model 6 and bootstrapping were uesed with a 95% confidence interval (CI).

3. Results

3.1. Participants' General and Disease-Related Characteristics

Participants' mean age was 52.47 years, with an average treatment duration of 34.5 months. Regarding their ability to perform activities at the time of the survey, 90 respondents (62.5%) were asymptomatic (able to perform activities as they did without the disease), and 54 respondents (37.5%) were symptomatic but fully mobile (e.g., light housework; Table 1).

Table 1. Characteristics of participants (N = 143).

Characteristic	Category	Mean (±SD) or n (%)
Age (years)		52.47 (±8.23)
Treatment period (months)		34.46 (±25.95)
Religious	Yes	80 (55.9%)
	No	63 (44.1%)
Employed	Yes	68 (47.6%)
	No	75 (52.4%)
Activity ability	Asymptomatic	89 (62.2%)
	Symptomatic but fully functional	54 (37.8%)

3.2. Correlations of Post-Traumatic Growth, Successful Aging, Resilience, and Intolerance of Uncertainty in Participants

Successful aging in this study was positively correlated with post-traumatic growth ($r = 0.708$, $p < 0.001$) and resilience ($r = 0.463$, $p < 0.001$), and negatively correlated with intolerance of uncertainty ($r = -0.282$, $p = 0.001$). Post-traumatic growth was positively correlated with resilience ($r = 0.318$. $p < 0.001$), and resilience was negatively correlated with intolerance of uncertainty ($r = -0.350$, $p < 0.001$). (Table 2).

Table 2. Correlations among variables (N = 143).

	Successful Aging	Post-Traumatic Growth	Resilience	Intolerance of Uncertainty
Post-traumatic growth	0.708 ***			
Resilience	0.463 ***	0.318 ***		
Intolerance of uncertainty	−0.282 ***	−0.155 (0.063)	−0.350 ***	1
Mean	2.71	3.38	2.99	2.31
SD	0.71	0.90	0.77	0.55

*** $p < 0.001$.

3.3. Mediating Effects of Resilience and Intolerance of Uncertainty on the Relationship between Post-Traumatic Growth and Successful Aging

Multicollinearity was examined prior to analyzing the mediating effect of resilience and intolerance of uncertainty on the relationship between post-traumatic growth and successful aging of participants. Subsequently, the tolerance limits were between 0.806 and 0.897, which was above 0.10; the variance of the inflation factor was between 1.115 and 1.240, which was below 10, indicating no problem with multicollinearity. Further, the Durbin–Watson index was 2.180, which was close to 2; the P-P plot showed a normal distribution, and the scatterplot of the standardized residuals confirmed homoscedasticity.

To test the mediating effect of resilience and intolerance of uncertainty on the relationship between post-traumatic growth and successful aging, religion, job, and activity ability, which showed significant differences in successful aging, were controlled and analyzed using the PROCESS macro model 6. Post-traumatic growth had a significant effect on the mediator resilience (B = 0.284, $p < 0.001$), and resilience had a significant effect on successful aging (B = 0.202, $p < 0.001$).

The direct effect for the successful aging of post-traumatic growth was 0.467 and was significant with a 95% bootstrap confidence interval (0.439 to 0.639) that did not include zero. The indirect effect of post-traumatic growth on successful aging, mediated by resilience, was 0.057, which was significant with a 95% bootstrap confidence interval (0.023 to 0.102) that did not include zero. The indirect effect of post-traumatic growth on successful aging, mediated by intolerance of uncertainty, was 0.006, which was not significant with a 95% bootstrap confidence interval (−0.009 to 0.027) that included zero. The indirect effect of post-traumatic growth on successful aging through both resilience and intolerance uncertainty was 0.009, which was also not significant with a 95% bootstrap confidence interval (−0.002 to 0.023) that included zero. (Table 3; Figure 1).

Table 3. Mediating effects of resilience and intolerance of uncertainty on post-traumatic growth and successful aging (N = 143).

	Unstandardized Coeff.	SE	95% CI (Lower)	95% CI (Upper)	Standardized Effect	p
Total effect	0.539	0.051	0.439	0.639	0.762	<0.001
Direct effect	0.467	0.050	0.368	0.566	0.661	<0.001
x → m1 → y	0.057	0.020	0.023	0.102	0.073	
x → m2 → y	0.006	0.009	−0.009	0.027	0.007	
x → m1 → m2 → y	0.009	0.007	−0.002	0.023	0.011	
Total indirect effect	0.072	0.024	0.029	0.122	0.092	

Note: Number of bootstrap samples for bias-corrected bootstrap confidence intervals; 5000. Level of confidence for all confidence intervals; 95%. x = post-traumatic growth; m1 = resilience, m2 = intolerance of uncertainty, y = successful aging.

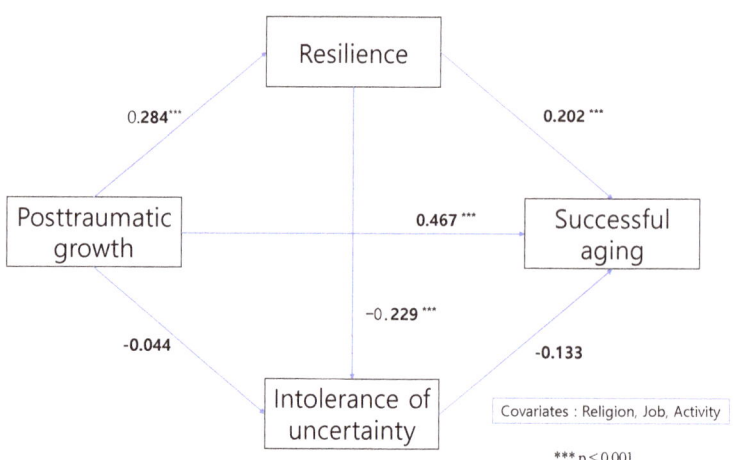

Figure 1. Mediating effects of resilience and intolerance of uncertainty on post-traumatic growth in successful aging.

4. Discussion

This study examined the mediating effects of resilience and intolerance of uncertainty on the relationship between post-traumatic growth and successful aging in breast cancer survivors. Our study provided several noteworthy findings that contribute to the understanding of these psychological constructs and their interplay in the context of successful aging.

One of the most salient findings is the mediating role of resilience in the relationship between post-traumatic growth and successful aging. Not only did post-traumatic growth significantly affect resilience, but resilience, significantly affected successful aging. This suggests that individuals who experience post-traumatic growth might foster a greater sense of resilience, which subsequently contributes to more successful aging.

Although direct comparisons of results were difficult owing to the lack of studies that comprehensively examined the relationship between these variables in patients with breast cancer, the current results supported previous research suggesting that post-traumatic growth [8,40] and resilience [41] influenced successful aging. An individual's resilience to cancer is the personal trait that protects him or herself against the disease and positively influences recovery [42]. Increased resilience to cancer promotes successful adaptation to one's condition. A previous study also reported that resilience to cancer was associated with positive mental health, quality of life, an improved pain threshold, increased physical activity, and improved rehabilitation outcomes in patients with cancer [43]. Promoting resilience focuses on interventions that address cognitive and problem-solving skills in stressful situations or focus on an individual's self-esteem or positive emotions to help him or her overcome negative situations by improving these internal characteristics [44]. Therefore, it is necessary to develop and apply programs to promote the resilience of patients with breast cancer through education on how to promote resilience, manage stress, and strengthen various internal characteristics of breast cancer survivors. Further, the findings indicate that as resilience increases, intolerance to uncertainty decreases. This is similar to previous research [21] that found a negative correlation between intolerance of uncertainty and resilience. Individuals with higher resilience are more likely to be resilient when faced with uncertainty and, thus feel less stress or anxiety about uncertainty as compared to their counterparts. This can occur through both direct and indirect effects, suggesting that increasing resilience can help improve one's ability to cope with uncertainty. Resilience could affect uncertainty tolerance through some mediating variables (e.g., self-efficacy and positive thinking). Hence, future research should explore which variables play this mediating role.

In contrast to resilience, intolerance of uncertainty did not play a significant mediating role in the relationship between post-traumatic growth and successful aging. This suggests that while intolerance of uncertainty could be relevant in other contexts, its role in the trajectory from post-traumatic growth to successful aging might be minimal or overshadowed by other more dominant factors, such as resilience. It was difficult to compare results with those of other studies, as research confirming the mediating effect of intolerance of uncertainty in the relationship between post-traumatic growth and successful aging was not available. However, this differed from the significant positive association between post-traumatic growth and intolerance of uncertainty in Jewish pregnant women [45] and from uncertainty acting as a significant barrier to successful aging in midlife [46]. Intolerance of uncertainty in breast cancer survivors could have had a lack of mediating effect on the relationship between post-traumatic growth and successful aging owing to a combination of factors, including individual characteristics and socio-psychological factors. Tolerance of uncertainty is a personality trait; people who have it can manage situations well in uncertainty without experiencing destructive anxiety [47]. Therefore, intolerance of uncertainty in breast cancer survivors could also affect many of the situations they experience. Further, since both post-traumatic growth and successful aging were negatively correlated with intolerance of uncertainty, future research should further examine the role of intolerance of uncertainty in the relationship between post-traumatic growth and successful aging.

Moreover, the role that negative variables, including depression and anxiety, along with intolerance of uncertainty, play in the relationship between post-traumatic growth and successful aging should be further explored.

Beyond the mediators, it is essential to acknowledge the direct impact of post-traumatic growth on successful aging. Our results indicate that even after accounting for the roles of resilience and intolerance of uncertainty, post-traumatic growth has a strong effect on successful aging. This was consistent with previous studies on post-traumatic growth that positively influenced successful aging in breast cancer survivors and middle-aged women [8,9]. Previous research has identified personal characteristics, disease factors, cognitive processes, coping strategies, social support, religion, spirituality, body roles, and physical activity as influencing post-traumatic growth in women with breast cancer [48]. This means that it is necessary to fully understand the post-traumatic growth of breast cancer survivors; develop and implement programs to support their post-traumatic growth and consequently help them age successfully; and consider the many variables that affect post-traumatic growth when developing programs to support post-traumatic growth. Future research will, therefore, need to identify which elements of post-traumatic growth are more important for successful aging.

Among the general characteristics and disease- and treatment-related characteristics of participants, the characteristics that made a significant difference in successful aging were "religion," "job," and "activity ability." Kim - and Kim [49] found significant differences in education level and job but not in the stage of cancer, time after surgery, type of surgery, chemotherapy, radiotherapy, targeted therapy, hormone therapy, or self-help groups for all disease-related characteristics among middle-aged breast cancer survivors. This was similar to previous research [8] that suggested that the loss of physical function or frailty in daily life did not have a direct effect on successful aging in breast cancer survivors. Coping processes, such as post-traumatic growth, contributed to successful aging rather than health status. Nevertheless, physical issues are important in aging, and biological factors and diseases have a significant impact on successful aging [50]. Therefore, in the future, it is necessary to confirm the relationship between each variable and successful aging in repeated studies with a larger sample size and patients with different types of cancer.

Limitations and future research Suggestions

This study was limited in the demographic variables that were collected, as well the ability to determine the response rate during the data collection phase. Data collection took place over a relatively short period. Participation in the survey was voluntary, which could, have resulted in unintended bias. This study only collected data from respondents from the Busan and Gyeongnam regions, and participants were outpatients at a single hospital. This could impact the generalizability of the results compared to the broader South Korean population. In addition, it did not reflect the relationship between the main variables and a wider range of variables (e.g., well-being, quality of life, depression, etc.), which should be considered in the future. This study can be used as a basis for identifying the extent of post-traumatic growth in breast cancer survivors and exploring ways to strengthen their resilience while developing nursing intervention programs to promote the successful aging of breast cancer survivors in clinical settings.

5. Conclusions

Successful aging among breast cancer survivors was positively correlated with post-traumatic growth and resilience and negatively correlated with intolerance of uncertainty. A mediating effect of resilience on the relationship between post-traumatic growth and successful aging was identified. There is a need to develop and apply intervention programs that consider post-traumatic growth and enhance resilience for successful aging in breast cancer survivors.

Author Contributions: Conceptualization, S.L. and K.S.K.; methodology, S.L. and H.L; software, S.J.Y.; validation, S.L. and H.L.; formal analysis, S.L., S.J.Y. and H.L; investigation, S.J.Y. and S.L.; resources, S.L. and K.S.K.; data curation, S.L., S.J.Y. and H.L.; writing—original draft preparation, S.L. and S.J.Y.; writing—review and editing, S.L. and H.L.; visualization, S.L., S.J.Y. and H.L.; supervision, S.L. and H.L.; project administration, S.L. and H.L. All authors have read and agreed to the published version of the manuscript.

Funding: This research received no external funding.

Institutional Review Board Statement: The study was conducted in accordance with the Declaration of Helsinki and approved by the Institutional Review Board of Kosin University Gospel Hospital in Gyeongsangnam-do (no. 2020-12-020) for studies involving humans.

Informed Consent Statement: Informed consent was obtained from all participants involved in the study.

Data Availability Statement: The data presented in this study are available on request from the corresponding author. The data are not publicly available owing to privacy restrictions.

Acknowledgments: The authors thank the study participants.

Conflicts of Interest: The authors declare no conflict of interest.

References

1. National Cancer Information Center. Main Contents [Internet]. Cancer in Statistics: Seoul, Republic of Korea, 2022. Available online: https://www.cancer.go.kr/ (accessed on 10 November 2022).
2. Korean Breast Cancer Society. Main Contents [Internet]. Breast Cancer: Seoul [White Paper]. 2022. Available online: https://www.kbcs.or.kr/journal/file/221018.pdf (accessed on 10 November 2022).
3. Jun, S.M. Successful Aging and Related Factors in Gastric Cancer Patients after Gastrectomy. Master's Thesis, Yonsei University, Seoul, Republic of Korea, 2013; pp. 1–79.
4. Flood, M. A mid-range nursing theory of successful aging. *J. Theory Constr. Test.* **2005**, *9*, 35–39.
5. Kozar-Westman, M.; Troutman-Jordan, M.; Nies, M.A. Successful aging among assisted living community older adult. *J. Nurs. Scholarsh.* **2013**, *45*, 238–246. [CrossRef] [PubMed]
6. Rowe, J.W.; Kahn, R.L. Successful aging. *Gerontologist* **1997**, *37*, 433–440. [CrossRef] [PubMed]
7. Syrowatka, A.; Motulsky, A.; Kurteva, S.; Hanley, J.A.; Dixon, W.G.; Meguerditchian, A.N.; Tamblyn, R. Predictors of distress in female breast cancer survivors: A systematic review. *Breast Cancer Res. Treat.* **2017**, *165*, 229–245. [CrossRef] [PubMed]
8. Yun, Y.H. Factors Influencing Successful Aging in Breast Cancer Survivors. Master's Thesis, Seoul National University, Seoul, Republic of Korea, 2020; pp. 1–103.
9. Vaishnavi, S.; Connor, K.; Davidson, J.R. An abbreviated version of the Connor-Davidson Resilience Scale (CD-RISC), the CD-RISC2: Psychometric properties and applications in psychopharmacological trials. *Psychiatry Res.* **2007**, *152*, 293–297. [CrossRef]
10. Joseph, S.; Linley, P.A.; Andrews, L.; Harris, G.; Howle, B.; Woodward, C.; Shevlin, M. Assessing positive and negative changes in the aftermath of adversity: Psychometric evaluation of the changes in outlook questionnaire. *Psychol. Assess.* **2005**, *17*, 70–80. [CrossRef] [PubMed]
11. Heo, C.M.; An, S.H. Relationship among subjective health, psychological well-being and successful aging of elderly participating in physical activity. *Korean J. Phys. Educ.* **2014**, *53*, 357–369.
12. Tedeschi, R.G.; Calhoun, L.G. Posttraumatic growth: Conceptual foundations and empirical evidence. *Psychol. Inq.* **2004**, *15*, 1–18. [CrossRef]
13. Liu, J.E.; Wang, H.Y.; Wang, M.L.; Su, Y.L.; Wang, P.L. Posttraumatic growth and psychological distress in Chinese early-stage breast cancer survivors: A longitudinal study. *Psycho-Oncology* **2014**, *23*, 437–443. [CrossRef]
14. Park, J.H.; Jung, Y.S.; Jung, Y.M. Factors influencing posttraumatic growth in survivors of breast cancer. *J. Korean Acad. Nurs.* **2016**, *46*, 454–462. [CrossRef]
15. Skaczkowski, G.; Hayman, T.; Strelan, P.; Miller, J.; Knott, V. Complementary medicine and recovery from cancer: The importance of post-traumatic growth. *Eur. J. Cancer Care (Engl.)* **2013**, *22*, 474–483. [CrossRef] [PubMed]
16. Kim, N.; Woo, Y.J. The effect of self-compassion, self-resilience and intolerance od uncertainty on job-seeking stress: For job seekers in the COVID-19 pandemic. *J. Learn.-Cent. Curric. Instr.* **2021**, *21*, 639–654. [CrossRef]
17. Choi, U.J.; Kim, Y.S.; Kang, J.S. Effect of uncertainty and resilience on stress for cancer patients. *Stress* **2018**, *26*, 250–256. [CrossRef]
18. Waugh, C.E.; Fredrickson, B.L.; Taylor, S.F. Adapting to life's slings and arrows: Individual differences in resilience when recovering from an anticipated threat. *J. Res. Pers.* **2008**, *42*, 1031–1046. [CrossRef] [PubMed]
19. Lee, H.J.; Jun, S.S. Factors related to posttraumatic growth in patients with colorectal cancer. *Korean J. Adult Nurs.* **2016**, *28*, 247–255. [CrossRef]
20. Wilson, B.A.; Morris, B.A.; Chambers, S. A structural equation model of posttraumatic growth after prostate cancer. *Psycho-Oncology* **2014**, *23*, 1212–1219. [CrossRef] [PubMed]

21. Nygren, B.; Aléx, L.; Jonsén, E.; Gustafson, Y.; Norberg, A.; Lundman, B. Resilience, sense of coherence, purpose in life and self-transcendence in relation to perceived physical and mental health among the oldest old. *Aging Ment. Health* **2005**, *9*, 354–362. [CrossRef] [PubMed]
22. Jeste, D.V.; Savla, G.N.; Thompson, W.K.; Vahia, I.V.; Glorioso, D.K.; Martin, A.S.; Palmer, B.W.; Rock, D.; Golshan, S.; Kraemer, H.C.; et al. Association between older age and more successful aging: Critical role of resilience and depression. *Am. J. Psychiatry* **2013**, *170*, 188–196. [CrossRef]
23. Shin, E.; Son, Y. The effects of intolerance of uncertainty on burnout among counselor: The mediating effect of self-compassion and burnout. *J. Humanit. Soc. Sci.* **2019**, *10*, 1091–1106. [CrossRef]
24. Lee, J.S. Effect of resilience on intolerance of uncertainty in nursing university students. *Nurs Forum* **2019**, *54*, 53–59. [CrossRef]
25. Freeston, M.H.; Rhéaume, J.; Letarte, H.; Dugas, M.J.; Ladouceur, R. Why do people worry? *Pers. Individ. Dif.* **1994**, *17*, 791–802. [CrossRef]
26. Buhr, K.; Dugas, M.J. The Intolerance of Uncertainty Scale: Psychometric properties of the English version. *Behav. Res. Ther.* **2002**, *40*, 931–945. [CrossRef] [PubMed]
27. Sexton, K.A.; Dugas, M.J. Defining distinct negative beliefs about uncertainty: Validating the factor structure of the intolerance of uncertainty scale. *Psychol. Assess.* **2009**, *21*, 176–186. [CrossRef] [PubMed]
28. Kurita, K.; Garon, E.B.; Stanton, A.L.; Meyerowitz, B.E. Uncertainty and psychological adjustment in patients with lung cancer. *Psycho-Oncology* **2013**, *22*, 1396–1401. [CrossRef] [PubMed]
29. Hill, E.M.; Hamm, A. Intolerance of uncertainty, social support, and loneliness in relation to anxiety and depressive symptoms among women diagnosed with ovarian cancer. *Psycho-Oncology* **2019**, *28*, 553–560. [CrossRef] [PubMed]
30. Taha, S.; Matheson, K.; Cronin, T.; Anisman, H. Intolerance of uncertainty, appraisals, coping, and anxiety: The case of the 2009 H1N1 pandemic. *Br. J. Health Psychol.* **2014**, *19*, 592–605. [CrossRef] [PubMed]
31. Jones, S.L.; Hadjistavropoulos, H.D.; Gullickson, K. Understanding health anxiety following breast cancer diagnosis. *Psychol. Health Med.* **2014**, *19*, 525–535. [CrossRef]
32. Antonovsky, A. *Health, Stress and Coping*; Jossey-Bass: San Francisco, CA, USA, 1979.
33. Antonovsky, A. *Unraveling the Mystery of Health*; Jossey-Bass: San Francisco, CA, USA, 1987.
34. Son, Y.J.; Song, E.K. Impact of health literacy on disease-related knowledge and adherence to self-care in patients with hypertension. *J. Korean Acad. Fundam. Nurs.* **2012**, *19*, 6–15. [CrossRef]
35. Kang, H.; Yeon, K.; Han, S.T. A review on the use of effect size in nursing research. *J. Korean Acad. Nurs.* **2015**, *45*, 641–649. [CrossRef]
36. Song, S.H.; Kim, K.H.; Lee, H.S.; Park, J.H. Validity and reliability of the Korean version of the posttraumatic growth inventory. *Korean J. Health Psychol.* **2009**, *14*, 193–214. [CrossRef]
37. Troutman, M.; Nies, M.A.; Small, S.; Bates, A. The development and testing of an instrument to measure successful aging. *Res. Gerontol. Nurs.* **2011**, *4*, 221–232. [CrossRef]
38. Jang, H.S. A Structural Equation Model for Successful Aging. Master's Thesis, Dankook University, Cheonan, Republic of Korea, 2016; pp. 1–124.
39. Choi, H.K. The dysfunctional effects of chronic worry and controllable-uncontrollable threats on problem-solving. *Korean J. Clin. Psychol.* **2003**, *22*, 287–302.
40. Kim, B.M. Perceptions of successful aging and the influencing factors in middle-aged women. *J. Korea Acad.-Ind. Coop. Soc.* **2018**, *19*, 91–99.
41. MacLeod, S.; Musich, S.; Hawkins, K.; Alsgaard, K.; Wicker, E.R. The impact of resilience among older adults. *Geriatr. Nurs.* **2016**, *37*, 266–272. [CrossRef] [PubMed]
42. Seiler, A.; Jenewein, J. Resilience in cancer patients. *Front. Psychiatry* **2019**, *10*, 208. [CrossRef] [PubMed]
43. Musich, S.; Wang, S.S.; Schaeffer, J.A.; Kraemer, S.; Wicker, E.; Yeh, C.S. The association of increasing resilience with positive health outcomes among older adults. *Geriatr. Nurs.* **2022**, *44*, 97–104. [CrossRef] [PubMed]
44. Kim, G.M.; Lim, J.Y.; Kim, E.J.; Park, S.M. Resilience of patients with chronic diseases: A systematic review. *Health Soc. Care Community* **2019**, *27*, 797–807. [CrossRef] [PubMed]
45. Chasson, M.; Taubman-Ben-Ari, O.; Abu-Sharkia, S. Posttraumatic growth in the wake of COVID-19 among Jewish and Arab pregnant women in Israel. *Psychol. Trauma* **2022**, *14*, 1324–1332. [CrossRef]
46. Subramaniam, V. Uncertainty and Successful Ageing: The Perspective from Malaysian Middle-Aged Adults Using Constructivist Grounded Theory. Ph.D. Thesis, The University of Edinburgh, Edinburgh, UK, 2019; pp. 1–421.
47. Kirzhetska, M.S.; Kirzhetskyy, Y.I.; Kohyt, Y.M.; Zelenko, N.M.; Zelenko, V.A.; Yaremkevych, R.V. Peculiarities of tolerance to uncertainty of people in late adulthood as a factor affecting mental well-being. *Wiad. Lek.* **2022**, *75*, 1839–1844. [CrossRef]
48. Zhai, J.; Newton, J.; Copnell, B. Posttraumatic growth experiences and its contextual factors in women with breast cancer: An integrative review. *Health Care Women Int.* **2019**, *40*, 554–580. [CrossRef]
49. Kim, E.J.; Kim, N. Comparison of perception of successful aging between late middle-aged breast cancer survivors and healthy women. *J. Korean Gerontol. Nurs.* **2017**, *19*, 48–56. [CrossRef]
50. Özsungur, F. Gerontechnological factors affecting successful aging of elderly. *Aging Male* **2020**, *23*, 520–532. [CrossRef]

Disclaimer/Publisher's Note: The statements, opinions and data contained in all publications are solely those of the individual author(s) and contributor(s) and not of MDPI and/or the editor(s). MDPI and/or the editor(s) disclaim responsibility for any injury to people or property resulting from any ideas, methods, instructions or products referred to in the content.

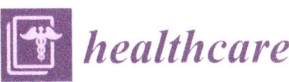

Article

Effects of Music on the Quality of Life of Family Caregivers of Terminal Cancer Patients: A Randomised Controlled Trial

Inmaculada Valero-Cantero [1], Cristina Casals [2,*], Milagrosa Espinar-Toledo [3], Francisco Javier Barón-López [4], Nuria García-Agua Soler [5] and María Ángeles Vázquez-Sánchez [6]

1. Puerta Blanca Clinical Management Unit, Malaga-Guadalhorce Health District, 29004 Malaga, Spain; inmaculada.valero.sspa@juntadeandalucia.es
2. ExPhy Research Group, Department of Physical Education, Instituto de Investigación e Innovación Biomédica de Cádiz (INiBICA), Universidad de Cádiz, 11519 Puerto Real, Spain
3. Rincón de la Victoria Clinical Management Unit, Malaga-Guadalhorce Health District, 29730 Malaga, Spain; milagrosa.espinar.sspa@juntadeandalucia.es
4. Department of Preventive Medicine, Public Health and Science History, Institute of Biomedical Research in Málaga (IBIMA), University of Malaga, 29007 Malaga, Spain; baron@uma.es
5. Department of Pharmacology, Faculty of Medicine, University of Malaga, 29010 Malaga, Spain; nuriags@uma.es
6. Department of Nursing, Faculty of Health Sciences, PASOS Research Group, UMA REDIAS Network of Law and Artificial Intelligence Applied to Health and Biotechnology, University of Malaga, 29071 Malaga, Spain; mavazquez@uma.es
* Correspondence: cristina.casals@uca.es; Tel.: +34-677180597

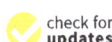

Citation: Valero-Cantero, I.; Casals, C.; Espinar-Toledo, M.; Barón-López, F.J.; García-Agua Soler, N.; Vázquez-Sánchez, M.Á. Effects of Music on the Quality of Life of Family Caregivers of Terminal Cancer Patients: A Randomised Controlled Trial. Healthcare 2023, 11, 1985. https://doi.org/10.3390/healthcare11141985

Academic Editor: Qiuping Li

Received: 3 June 2023
Revised: 6 July 2023
Accepted: 7 July 2023
Published: 9 July 2023

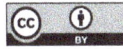

Copyright: © 2023 by the authors. Licensee MDPI, Basel, Switzerland. This article is an open access article distributed under the terms and conditions of the Creative Commons Attribution (CC BY) license (https://creativecommons.org/licenses/by/4.0/).

Abstract: The aim of this study was to investigate the effects of listening to self-chosen music on the quality of life of family caregivers of cancer patients receiving palliative home care. A total of 82 family caregivers were assigned either to the intervention group ($n = 41$) or to the control group ($n = 41$) in this double-blind, multicentre, randomised controlled clinical trial. The recruitment period was between July 2020 and September 2021. The intervention group received individualised pre-recorded music in daily 30 min sessions for 7 consecutive days. The control group was given a recorded repetition of the basic therapeutic training education also in 30 min sessions for 7 consecutive days. The primary endpoint assessed was the caregivers' quality of life (Quality of Life Family Version and European Quality of Life visual analogue scale) before and after the intervention. The secondary endpoint was their perceived satisfaction with the intervention (Client Satisfaction Questionnaire). The music intervention was successful, producing a tangible improvement in the caregivers' quality of life ($p < 0.01$) and satisfaction with the care provided ($p = 0.002$). The intervention was not only effective but produced no adverse effects. This study encourages the use of self-chosen music as a complementary intervention in nursing care for family caregivers of palliative cancer patients.

Keywords: informal caregivers; complementary therapy; alternative therapy; palliative care; self-reported quality of life; self-perceived quality of life; client satisfaction; music medicine

1. Introduction

Globally, cancer represents the second most common cause of death, with a staggering death toll of nearly ten million individuals in 2020 [1]. Prompt and effective palliative care can help manage physical symptoms as well as psychological and spiritual distress, improving patients' quality of life and potentially prolonging survival. Patients with advanced cancer need palliative care as early as possible [2], which is typically administered at home, as it is often the preferred setting for patients to receive care while remaining in their social environment and while also minimizing the burden on hospital resources [3,4]. Therefore, home-based palliative care plays a critical role in comprehensive cancer care, providing patients with a supportive and comforting environment for receiving end-of-life care.

Home-based palliative care has demonstrated promising results in reducing hospital readmissions and healthcare costs. Despite the fact that palliative care is typically provided by healthcare professionals, including nurses, physicians, and social workers, who work together to manage patients' symptoms and address their physical, emotional, and spiritual needs, home-based palliative care can be provided by health professionals but also relies on the essential contribution of one or more caregivers, usually family members, who provide social support and round-the-clock care with no financial compensation [5,6].

These functions—proving care and companionship for a person at the end of their life—often provoke major alterations in the caregiver, such as anxiety, fatigue, and an intense sensation of overload [7–9] together with depression [10], sleep disturbances [11], and impaired quality of life overall [12,13]. Supporting caregivers in the context of home-based palliative care is therefore crucial to ensure that both the patient and the caregiver receive the best possible care and support during this difficult time. Addressing caregivers' well-being can contribute to more sustainable and successful home-based palliative care delivery. Therefore, it is essential to understand the unique challenges faced by caregivers in the context of home-based palliative care and to develop effective interventions to support them.

In this regard, the significance of addressing the quality of life of family caregivers of patients with cancer in palliative care is underscored. The parameter "quality of life" is composed of different domains reflecting an individual's general level of health and well-being. It can be measured using dimensions with physical, psychological, social, and spiritual components [14]. For caregivers of patients in palliative care, their quality of life is often reduced by alterations such as overload [15] and the absence of necessary support [13]. In accordance with the indications of the World Health Organization, palliative care is provided to alleviate symptoms and to enhance the patient's quality of life [16]. During home-based palliative care, interventions should also be conducted to assure caregivers' own quality of life, helping them provide optimum levels of care [17,18].

One such intervention may be that of psychoeducation [19], which refers to any structured psychological educational program. However, despite the acknowledged importance of assuring caregivers' quality of life, few studies have been conducted to determine the effectiveness of this and related interventions [17]. One example is music medicine, which is defined as "when medical or health personnel offer pre-recorded music for passive listening" [20]. This is a complementary musical intervention, which is defined as "a group of diverse medical and health care systems, practices, and products that are not generally considered part of conventional medicine" [21]. Regarding listening to music, auditory signals are an important aspect of human sensory systems. Among them, music has a special capacity that is capable of inspiring emotions. The temporal limbic system, formed, among other structures, by the amygdala, the hippocampus, the ventral and dorsal striata, and the auditory cortex, helps decode the emotional value of the music heard [22].

Music may both create emotions and alter moods [22,23]. For this reason, listening to music is sometimes used as a complement in the care of patients with cancer to improve fatigue, depression, and sleep and decrease pain, among other symptoms [24–26]. However, this benefit has not been demonstrated in all the symptoms studied, and therefore, more studies are required in this regard [27]. Focusing on caregivers of patients with advanced cancer, it has been previously shown that music has benefits on symptoms of anxiety, fatigue, depression, and blood volume pulse amplitude [28,29]. However, despite the importance of quality of life as a health indicator, to our knowledge, no previous clinical trials have been performed to evaluate the advantages of music for family caregivers of palliative-care patients in the home [30].

The aim of the present study is to investigate the potential benefits of a complementary music medicine intervention for the family caregivers of patients in palliative home care. Our main study hypothesis was that the intervention group would achieve a greater improvement in quality of life than the control group after the seven-day intervention. The secondary hypothesis was that the intervention group would also report greater satisfaction than the control group with the therapy received.

2. Materials and Methods

2.1. Design

To address the previous hypotheses, we conducted a double-blind, multicentre, randomised controlled clinical trial of family caregivers for cancer patients in palliative home care [31]. The intervention group received a complementary music medicine intervention for seven consecutive days, while the control group received conventional treatment also for seven consecutive days. Both groups were assessed for quality of life and satisfaction with therapy at baseline and after the intervention period. The study is registered at Clinical Trials.gov, reference code: NCT04052074; registered on 9 August 2019.

We recently published a scientific article of this short-term trial [32], suggesting that using self-chosen music significantly reduced caregiver burden among family caregivers of patients with advanced cancer. While burden focuses on the negative aspects of caregiving, such as the level of strain, stress, and disruptions to the caregiver's life, quality of life provides a broader perspective that includes positive aspects, such as personal fulfilment, social support, and the caregiver's ability to find meaning in their caregiving role. Burden is often related to the objective demands of caregiving, such as the intensity of care required, financial strain, and time commitments. Quality of life, on the other hand, reflects the caregiver's subjective appraisal of their well-being, encompassing physical health, emotional well-being, social functioning, and overall life satisfaction.

Therefore, the present manuscript specifically presents the quality-of-life results of this clinical trial since it allows for a clearer and more focused presentation of findings. This level of depth and granularity enhances the scientific understanding of each variable and contributes to the overall body of knowledge in the field.

2.2. Participants

The study participants were all family caregivers for cancer patients in palliative home care, recruited at six primary-care clinical management units within the Malaga-Guadalhorce Health District from Andalusia, Spain. The participants were recruited by reference to the lists of patients included in the Palliative Care Assistance Process in the DIRAYA Digital Health Record maintained at each of the above units, using convenience sampling. The following inclusion criteria were applied: (i) family caregiver; (ii) age at least 18 years. Any caregivers with severe hearing loss preventing them from using an mp3 device or mobile phone were excluded from the study group.

2.3. Research Ethics

This clinical trial underwent a comprehensive ethical review process and was granted approval by the Research Ethics Committee of the Province of Malaga on 28 March 2019 (reference code: AP-0157-2018). The study adhered to the principles outlined in the Declaration of Helsinki, which ensures the protection of participants' rights, welfare, and privacy during research studies. All participants were provided with detailed information regarding the objectives, procedures, and potential risks and benefits of the study, both verbally and in writing, and gave prior signed informed consent.

2.4. Measures

The main outcome was the caregivers' quality of life, which was assessed using the following scales:

- The Quality of Life Family Version (QOL-FV) 14, validated in Spanish [33], which measures the quality of life of family caregivers for patients with cancer, consists of thirty-seven items, scored on a scale ranging from 0 = worst result to 10 = best result (although several are coded by means of an inverse score). The instrument has four

sub-scales or domains: physical well-being, psychological well-being, social concerns, and spiritual well-being;
- The European Quality of Life—5 dimensions (EuroQol-5D-5L) questionnaire was developed in the United Kingdom and in Spain [34]. The questionnaire score is obtained using a visual analogue scale, ranging from 0 to 100, representing "worst imaginable state of health" to "best imaginable state of health", respectively.

Moreover, the secondary outcome was the caregivers' satisfaction with the intervention, and it was assessed using the Client Satisfaction Questionnaire (CSQ-8) [35], validated in Spanish [36]. This self-administered questionnaire consists of eight questions scored on a 4-point Likert-type scale (in four cases, the score is inverse). The final assessment is obtained by summing these scores and can range from 8 to 32 points.

2.5. Sample Size and Randomisation

The necessary sample size was calculated according to the method described by Hanser et al. [37], assuming a standard deviation of 1.23 for satisfaction, a power of 80%, and an alpha error of 5%. Furthermore, an increase of one point in caregiver satisfaction was considered relevant. Under these premises, the study required two samples of 34 caregivers. To allow for a possible dropout rate of 20%, this sample size was increased to two samples of 41 caregivers.

The randomisation of the participants between the control and intervention groups was carried out as follows. Cards were marked "Intervention group" or "Control group" and inserted into sealed opaque envelopes, which were then shuffled and numbered. Each participant was assigned a number by order of enrolment. The researcher performing the randomisation then opened the envelope corresponding to each number in turn and assigned the participant accordingly. In this double-blind trial, therefore, neither the caregivers nor the evaluators knew the group to which each participant belonged.

2.6. Intervention, Control Group, and Masking

All participants received conventional health care before the intervention in same conditions with basic therapeutic education for palliative care, which is part of the regular health care service in our health centres and is provided by nurses.

Then, the caregivers in the intervention group received, apart from the mentioned conventional health care, a music medicine intervention using pre-recorded music provided via an mp3 device or mobile phone. The music used was individualised, chosen by each participant to ensure that the music enhanced their well-being. The intervention consisted of a 30 min music session received daily for seven days. The caregiver was instructed not to perform any other activity during the session.

The participants in the control group received the conventional health care, and in addition, in order to mask the fact of their belonging to the control group (both to the participants and to the evaluators), they received a recorded repetition of this conventional treatment using an mp3 device or mobile phone. This activity was also performed in 30 min sessions received daily for seven consecutive days.

All study participants and clinical trial evaluators were blinded to the participants' membership of the control or the intervention group. The study assessments were carried out by the case-manager nurses of the respective primary-care clinical management units.

2.7. Data Collection and Analyses

The study data were compiled between July 2020 and September 2021 at interviews during home visits and via self-administered questionnaires. If any caregiver had difficulty understanding or responding to the questionnaire items, they were helped by the corresponding case-management nurse. Data on the participants' quality of life for both the control and the intervention groups were assessed before the intervention and seven days later after its conclusion. Their satisfaction was also assessed at this second time point.

The primary outcomes considered were the changes in the QOL-FV and EuroQol-5D-5L scores, between the baseline and the endpoint, and the outcomes achieved by the members of the control group with respect to those in the intervention group.

The secondary outcome considered was the participants' satisfaction with the intervention as assessed using CSQ-8 for the control group in comparison with the intervention group.

The inter-group comparisons of the questionnaire scores obtained were made using the non-parametric Mann–Whitney test. Moreover, the groups were separately analysed comparing the pre-post differences with respect to 0 by applying a one-sample Wilcoxon test. The quantitative variables are expressed as medians, means, and standard deviations. A two-sided p-value < 0.05 was considered statistically significant. All data analyses were performed using SPSS version 23.0 statistical software on an intention-to-treat basis.

3. Results

Results were obtained from all 82 participants. No adverse events were reported, and all participants completed the full programme. The flow diagram for the study is presented in Figure 1. Regarding baseline characteristics, there were no significant differences between the two groups (Table 1). The following change-from-baseline results were obtained: intervention vs. control group for the EuroQol-5D-5L: 6.29 (10.71)/−3.76 (7.26), $p < 0.001$; total QOL-FV: 0.16 (0.75)/−0.35 (0.94), $p = 0.008$; CSQ-8 final score: 27.54 (3.25)/24.80 (4.03), $p = 0.002$ (see Table 2).

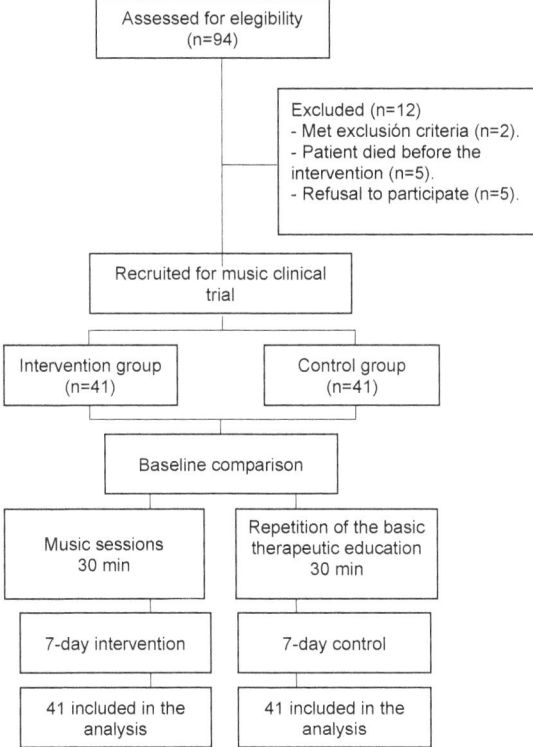

Figure 1. Flowchart of the study.

Table 1. Socio-demographic characteristics of caregivers.

	Total (n = 82)	Intervention Group (n = 41)	Control Group (n = 41)	p-Value
Age (years)	62.71 (12.56)	63.12 (12.81)	62.31 (12.46)	0.626
Sex				
Female	72 (87.8%)	34 (82.9%)	38 (92.7%)	0.177
Male	10 (12.2%)	7 (17.1%)	3 (7.3%)	
Education				
No formal education	11 (13.4%)	5 (12.2%)	6 (14.6%)	
Primary	39 (47.6%)	21 (51.2%)	18 (43.9%)	1.000
Secondary	22 (26.8%)	10 (24.4%)	12 (29.3%)	
University	10 (12.2%)	5 (12.2%)	5 (9.8%)	
Relationship to the person cared for				
Spouse	47 (57.3%)	27 (65.9%)	20 (48.8%)	
Daughter/son	25 (30.5%)	8 (19.5%)	17 (41.5%)	0.101
Other	10 (12.2%)	6 (14.6%)	4 (9.8%)	
Hours of daily care	17.47 (7.14)	18.07 (6.98)	16.87 (7.34)	0.448
VAS of the EuroQol-5D-5L	82.61 (14.79)	81.71 (15.99)	83.51 (13.63)	0.694
QOL-FV (scores)				
Physical well-being	7.08 (2.46)	7.12 (2.42)	7.04 (2.53)	0.948
Psychological well-being	5.56 (1.51)	5.42 (1.62)	5.71 (1.38)	0.649
Social concerns	5.95 (1.93)	5.91 (2.04)	6.00 (1.83)	0.981
Spiritual wellness	3,98 (1,81)	4.17 (1.85)	3.79 (1.78)	0.452
Total QOL-FV	5.64 (1.43)	5.65 (1.58)	5.63 (1.28)	0.742

Results are presented as mean (standard deviation) or numbers (%). p-value corresponds to the Mann–Whitney U-test, except for sex (chi-squared test) and education (Fisher's exact test). VAS of the EuroQol-5D-5L, visual analogue scale of the European Quality of Life—5 dimensions; QOL-FV, Quality of Life Family Version.

Table 2. Outcomes differences between groups before and after the 7-day intervention.

	Intervention Group				Control Group				p-Value between Groups
	Pre	Post	Change	p-Value	Pre	Post	Change	p-Value	
QOL-FV (scores)									
Physical well-being	7.12 (2.47)	7.56 (1.84)	0.44 (1.70)	**0.006**	7.04 (2.53)	6.18 (2.34)	−0.86 (1.89)	0.106	**0.004**
Psychological well-being	5.42 (1.67)	5.63 (1.58)	0.22 (1.00)	0.297	5.71 (1.39)	5.53 (1.60)	−0.18 (1.09)	0.272	0.119
Social concerns	5.91 (2.04)	6.19 (1.84)	0.28 (1.03)	0.233	6.00 (1.83)	5.69 (2.04)	−0.31 (1.62)	0.065	**0.024**
Spiritual wellness	4.17 (1.85)	3.97 (1.54)	−0.30 (1.27)	0.825	3.79 (1.78)	3.76 (1.85)	−0.03 (1.00)	0.196	0.883
Total QOL-FV	5.65 (1.58)	5.81 (1.23)	0.16 (0.75)	**0.023**	5.63 (1.28)	5.28 (1.25)	−0.35 (0.94)	0.102	**0.008**
VAS of the EuroQol-5D-5L	81.71 (15.99)	88.00 (13.03)	6.29 (10.71)	**0.002**	83.51 (13.63)	79.76 (12.1)	−3.76 (7.26)	**0.001**	**<0.001**
CSQ-8 (score)	-	27.54 (3.25)	-	-	-	24.80 (4.03)	-	-	**0.002**

p-value corresponds to pre-post differences respect to 0 in the Wilcoxon test, while p-value between groups corresponds to control group change versus that of the intervention group in the Mann–Whitney U-test. All p-values < 0.05 are presented in bold. VAS, visual analogue scale; CSQ-8, Client Satisfaction Questionnaire.

4. Discussion

This clinical trial was undertaken to investigate the benefits of music in relation to the quality of life reported by family caregivers of cancer patients in palliative home care and to determine these caregivers' satisfaction with the health care provided. The study results reveal a significant improvement in the quality of life reported and increased satisfaction with the health care provided.

The caregivers of palliative-care patients normally experience a worsening quality of life as the disease progresses [38], even in 7 days [39]. Although a previous study found no significant difference in quality of life for caregivers who listened to music [28], our clinical trial did reveal such an improvement according to the total QOL-FV scores obtained by the intervention group. This difference may be due to the fact that the previous study was quasi-experimental [28]. Moreover, the music used was that recommended by the authors, while our clinical trial used the caregivers' own choices of music.

Our analysis of the results for the four QOL-FV subscales reflect improved physical well-being and social concerns following the music intervention. However, there were no significant differences for the spiritual scale, indicating that although music medicine seems to enhance the quality of life in general, it does not have this effect regarding spiritual/religious aspects. A previous study conducted on another continent highlighted spiritual support as a need for family caregivers of cancer patients [40]. This finding may be related to the participants' faith (or lack of it) and/or its possible loss due to the disease process experienced [41]. More studies are encouraged, as a review article concluded that studies of psychosocial interventions aimed at improving the quality of life of both cancer patients and their family caregivers pay relatively little attention to spiritual well-being [42]. In addition, although the intervention group reported improved psychological well-being in our study, there was no significant difference in this respect compared to the control group.

The above findings, referring to the results obtained with the QOL-FV scale, were corroborated by the evaluation based on the EuroQol-5D-5L scale, which, among other items, concerns the "quality of life today". The congruent results obtained through the utilization of two distinct scales provide support for our research hypothesis, which posits that the implementation of self-chosen music interventions can enhance the quality of life experienced by family caregivers of cancer patients undergoing palliative care in a home setting.

In addition to addressing the study hypotheses, the potential practical applications of our findings are significant. The positive results seen in the intervention group highlight the potential for complementary music interventions to be used as a valuable tool in improving the quality of life and satisfaction of family caregivers in the context of home-based palliative care. The cancer-survivorship care plan should thoroughly acknowledge the intricate and enduring impact of unaddressed caregiver needs on their distinct dimensions of quality of life [43]. This could ultimately lead to better experiences for both caregivers and patients while reducing the burden on healthcare resources. Thus, the potential for widespread adoption and implementation in clinical settings is encouraged.

Indeed, we previously proposed this complementary music intervention as a useful strategy to reduce caregiver burden among these participants, suggesting its potential as a short-term relief strategy in family caregivers of palliative-care cancer patients [32]. However, the relationship between burden and quality of life is not consistent. As is shown in Table A1, the caregivers' burden was statistically associated only with the VAS of the EuroQol-5D-5L (moderate relationship), without significant associations with any subscale or the total score of the QOL-FV. The absence of a statistically significant relationship between the caregivers' burden and their quality of life is due to the fact that both concepts differ [44]. On the one hand, caregiver burden can be defined as the distress that caregivers feel as a result of providing care due to their caregiving responsibilities. It encompasses various aspects, such as the demands of providing care, financial difficulties, disruption of daily routines, and emotional distress. On the other hand, quality of life refers to the subjective well-being and satisfaction in various domains of life, including physical, psychological, social, and spiritual aspects [44].

Therefore, interventions aimed at supporting family caregivers should not only address the reduction of caregiver burden but also focus on improving their quality of life. These interventions may include self-chosen music sessions [45]. In the context of family caregivers of cancer patients, maintaining and enhancing their quality of life is of paramount importance to ensure their well-being and ability to continue providing effective care. Our study adds to the growing body of literature on the effectiveness of complementary therapies in healthcare, particularly in the context of palliative care, and highlights the potential for further research and development of such interventions. The practical applications of our findings underscore the importance of incorporating complementary therapies into traditional nursing care, particularly for those caring for terminally ill patients at home, in order to provide comprehensive and holistic support to their caregivers.

Another aspect studied is that of the caregivers' satisfaction with the care received. This question is important because it is not sufficient for a novel intervention to produce an objective improvement; it must also be considered appropriate, agreeable, and useful by those for whom it is intended since the success of any such intervention depends on the participants' cooperation and adherence. There are many determinants of satisfaction with health care, but the positive signs indicated in our study suggest that the musical medicine intervention was beneficial to the participants' physical and mental health [46]. This conclusion is corroborated by the fact that the caregivers in the intervention group were significantly more satisfied with the care received than those in the control group.

These findings highlight the potential for complementary musical interventions to enhance overall patient and caregiver experiences in the context of home-based palliative care, ultimately leading to improved quality of life and outcomes for those receiving care. Further research is necessary to explore the full range of potential applications and benefits, ultimately paving the way for the integration of these interventions into standard care practices and ensuring the delivery of comprehensive palliative care as well as in different settings and populations.

While the results of our clinical trial have provided novel and promising findings, it is important to acknowledge certain limitations that may affect the generalizability and long-term implications of our findings. First, one limitation is that our study sample consisted of participants recruited solely from public health clinics. Moreover, they were all located in urban areas. For both of these reasons, our findings may not reflect the experiences and outcomes of individuals utilizing private healthcare systems or those residing in rural areas, and therefore, caution should be exercised when generalising our results to broader populations. Consequently, the generalisability of our results may be limited. To address this limitation, future research should aim to investigate the effectiveness of complementary musical interventions in diverse populations, including individuals from various cultural backgrounds. By examining the impact of these interventions across different settings and demographics, a deeper comprehensive understanding of the potential impact of these interventions and the development of tailored approaches to meet the specific needs of different populations could be achieved.

Second, an aspect to consider is the durability of the effects observed in our study. It has not been established whether the effectiveness of music medicine persists over time or whether other similar interventions employed on a regular basis would be equally useful. Furthermore, the control group in this study underwent a repetition of the standard treatment consisting of varying 30 min sessions conducted over a 7-day period. Notably, participants were informed in advance by a nurse about this arrangement. This blinded design was implemented to address internal validity concerns, as it is known that receiving additional attention or care can positively influence quality of life and satisfaction with received care. However, it is crucial to acknowledge that the recorded conventional treatment itself may have influenced participants' quality of life. Consequently, future studies should consider comparing different conditions and groups to obtain a more comprehensive understanding of the topic. Therefore, further studies could compare different conditions and groups to provide a more comprehensive understanding. Nevertheless, the method we describe was applied very rigorously, and it can be replicated without difficulty.

Finally, a notable constraint of this study lies in the temporal scope of the intervention, which is confined to a mere 7-day period. Further research is needed to investigate the long-term effectiveness of self-chosen music sessions and to compare it with other similar interventions that could be integrated into routine care.

5. Conclusions

The intervention group exhibited a significant improvement in quality of life compared to the control group, indicating that the intervention positively impacted their overall well-being. Additionally, the intervention group reported higher levels of satisfaction with the therapy received, suggesting a positive subjective experience. In conclusion, the results of our study provide evidence to support the use of complementary musical interventions in the context of home-based palliative care for family caregivers of terminally ill patients.

Our intervention was shown to be highly effective, producing significant improvements in both the quality of life and satisfaction with care of participants without any reported adverse effects. The positive outcomes seen in our study highlight the potential benefits of incorporating complementary therapies into traditional nursing care, particularly for those caring for terminally ill patients at home. By incorporating music as a complementary intervention, we can address their emotional, psychological, spiritual, and social well-being.

Future research is needed to further explore the potential applications and benefits of such interventions in different populations and settings. In addition, it is encouraged to thoroughly analyse the potential long-term effects of such interventions to ensure their sustained efficacy in the context of home-based palliative care and also to corroborate whether the implementation of complementary musical interventions in nursing care could ultimately lead to improved outcomes and experiences for both patients and their caregivers.

Author Contributions: Conceptualization, I.V.-C., C.C. and M.Á.V.-S.; methodology, I.V.-C. and M.Á.V.-S.; software, F.J.B.-L.; formal analysis, F.J.B.-L.; investigation, I.V.-C., M.E.-T., N.G.-A.S. and M.Á.V.-S.; resources, I.V.-C., C.C. and M.Á.V.-S.; data curation, I.V.-C., F.J.B.-L. and M.Á.V.-S.; writing—original draft preparation, I.V.-C., C.C. and M.Á.V.-S.; writing—review and editing, M.E.-T., F.J.B.-L. and N.G.-A.S.; supervision, M.Á.V.-S.; project administration, I.V.-C.; funding acquisition, I.V.-C., C.C. and M.Á.V.-S. All authors have read and agreed to the published version of the manuscript.

Funding: This research was funded externally, involving research, development, and innovation (R + D + I) in biomedical and health sciences in Andalusia (Spain), obtained from the Regional Health Ministry of "Junta de Andalucia", grant numbers AP-0157-2018 and AP-0225-2019.

Institutional Review Board Statement: The study was conducted in accordance with the Declaration of Helsinki and approved by the Research Ethics Committee of the Province of Malaga on 28 March 2019 (File number: AP-0157-2018, 0638-N-18).

Informed Consent Statement: Informed consent was obtained from all subjects involved in the study.

Data Availability Statement: Study data are available on reasonable request to the corresponding author.

Conflicts of Interest: The authors declare no conflict of interest.

Appendix A

Table A1. Regression analysis between the Caregiver Strain Index and the quality of life of family caregivers of palliative cancer patients.

	B	Standard Error	β	*p*-Value
VAS of the EuroQol-5D-5L	−0.082	0.020	−0.401	0.001

Dependent variable: Caregiver Strain Index. Excluded variables: Total score of the Quality of Life Family Version and the subscales physical well-being, psychological well-being, social concerns, and spiritual wellness. VAS of the EuroQol-5D-5L, visual analogue scale of the European Quality of Life—5 dimensions.

References

1. Ferlay, J.; Ervik, M.; Lam, F.; Colombet, M.; Mery, L.; Piñeros, M. *Global Cancer Observatory: Cancer Today*; International Agency for Research on Cancer: Lyon, France, 2020. Available online: https://gco.iarc.fr/today (accessed on 10 February 2022).
2. Kaasa, S.; Loge, J.H.; Aapro, M.; Albreht, T.; Anderson, R.; Bruera, E.; Brunelli, C.; Caraceni, A.; Cervantes, A.; Currow, D.C.; et al. Integration of oncology and palliative care: A Lancet Oncology Commission. *Lancet Oncol.* **2018**, *19*, e588–e653. [CrossRef] [PubMed]
3. Shepperd, S.; Gonçalves-Bradley, D.C.; Straus, S.E.; Wee, B. Hospital at home: Home-based end-of-life care. *Cochrane Database Syst. Rev.* **2021**, *2021*, CD009231. [CrossRef]
4. Woodman, C.; Baillie, J.; Sivell, S. The preferences and perspectives of family caregivers towards place of care for their relatives at the end-of-life. A systematic review and thematic synthesis of the qualitative evidence. *BMJ Support. Palliat. Care* **2016**, *6*, 418–429. [CrossRef] [PubMed]
5. Kelly, E.P.; Meara, A.; Hyer, M.; Payne, N.; Pawlik, T.M. Understanding the Type of Support Offered Within the Caregiver, Family, and Spiritual/Religious Contexts of Cancer Patients. *J. Pain Symptom Manag.* **2019**, *58*, 56–64. [CrossRef]
6. Alvariza, A.; Häger-Tibell, L.; Holm, M.; Steineck, G.; Kreicbergs, U. Increasing preparedness for caregiving and death in family caregivers of patients with severe illness who are cared for at home—Study protocol for a web-based intervention. *BMC Palliat. Care* **2020**, *19*, 33–38. [CrossRef]
7. Perpiñá-Galvañ, J.; Orts-Beneito, N.; Fernández-Alcántara, M.; García-Sanjuán, S.; García-Caro, M.P.; Cabañero-Martínez, M.J. Level of Burden and Health-Related Quality of Life in Caregivers of Palliative Care Patients. *Int. J. Environ. Res. Public Health* **2019**, *16*, 4806. [CrossRef]
8. Lv, X.-Q.; Liu, J.-J.; Feng, Y.; Li, S.-W.; Qiu, H.; Hong, J.-F. Predictive model of psychological distress in family caregivers of patients with cancer: A cross-sectional study. *Support. Care Cancer* **2021**, *29*, 5091–5101. [CrossRef]
9. El-Jawahri, A.; Greer, J.A.; Park, E.R.; Jackson, V.A.; Kamdar, M.; Rinaldi, S.P.; Gallagher, E.R.; Jagielo, A.D.; Topping, C.E.; Elyze, M.; et al. Psychological Distress in Bereaved Caregivers of Patients With Advanced Cancer. *J. Pain Symptom Manag.* **2021**, *61*, 488–494. [CrossRef]
10. Govina, O.; Vlachou, E.; Kalemikerakis, I.; Papageorgiou, D.; Kavga, A.; Konstantinidis, T. Factors Associated with Anxiety and Depression among Family Caregivers of Patients Undergoing Palliative Radiotherapy. *Asia-Pac. J. Oncol. Nurs.* **2019**, *6*, 283–291. [CrossRef]
11. Valero-Cantero, I.; Wärnberg, J.; Carrión-Velasco, Y.; Martínez-Valero, F.J.; Casals, C.; Vázquez-Sánchez, M. Predictors of sleep disturbances in caregivers of patients with advanced cancer receiving home palliative care: A descriptive cross-sectional study. *Eur. J. Oncol. Nurs.* **2021**, *51*, 101907. [CrossRef]
12. Oechsle, K.; Ullrich, A.; Marx, G.; Benze, G.; Wowretzko, F.; Zhang, Y.; Dickel, L.-M.; Heine, J.; Wendt, K.N.; Nauck, F.; et al. Prevalence and Predictors of Distress, Anxiety, Depression, and Quality of Life in Bereaved Family Caregivers of Patients With Advanced Cancer. *Am. J. Hosp. Palliat. Med.* **2019**, *37*, 201–213. [CrossRef] [PubMed]
13. Norinder, M.; Årestedt, K.; Lind, S.; Axelsson, L.; Grande, G.; Ewing, G.; Holm, M.; Öhlén, J.; Benkel, I.; Alvariza, A. Higher levels of unmet support needs in spouses are associated with poorer quality of life—A descriptive cross-sectional study in the context of palliative home care. *BMC Palliat. Care* **2021**, *20*, 132. [CrossRef] [PubMed]
14. Ferrell, B.R.; Wisdom, C.; Wenzl, C. Quality of life as an outcome variable in the management of cancer pain. *Cancer* **1989**, *63*, 2321–2327. [CrossRef] [PubMed]
15. Tan, J.-Y.; Molassiotis, A.; Lloyd-Williams, M.; Yorke, J. Burden, emotional distress and quality of life among informal caregivers of lung cancer patients: An exploratory study. *Eur. J. Cancer Care* **2018**, *27*, e12691. [CrossRef]
16. World Health Organization. *Integrated Health Services, Quality of Care. Quality Health Services and Palliative Care: Practical Approaches and Resources to Support Policy, Strategy and Practice*; World Health Organization: Geneva, Switzerland, 2021; ISBN 978-92-4-003516-4. Available online: https://www.who.int/publications/i/item/9789240035164 (accessed on 10 February 2022).
17. Sun, V.; Raz, D.J.; Kim, J.Y. Caring for the informal cancer caregiver. *Curr. Opin. Support. Palliat. Care* **2019**, *13*, 238–242. [CrossRef]
18. Litzelman, K.; Kent, E.E.; Mollica, M.; Rowland, J.H. How Does Caregiver Well-Being Relate to Perceived Quality of Care in Patients With Cancer? Exploring Associations and Pathways. *J. Clin. Oncol.* **2016**, *34*, 3554–3561. [CrossRef]

19. Treanor, C.J. Psychosocial support interventions for cancer caregivers: Reducing caregiver burden. *Curr. Opin. Support. Palliat. Care* **2020**, *14*, 247–262. [CrossRef] [PubMed]
20. Dileo, C. A classification model for music and medicine. In *Applications of Music in Medicine*; National Association of Music Therapy: Washington, DC, USA, 1999; pp. 1–6.
21. National Center for Complementary and Integrative Health (NCCIH). Complementary, Alternative, or Integrative Health: What's in A Name? 2021. Available online: http://nccam.nih.gov/health/whatiscam (accessed on 10 February 2022).
22. Koelsch, S. A coordinate-based meta-analysis of music-evoked emotions. *Neuroimage* **2020**, *223*, 117350. [CrossRef] [PubMed]
23. Koelsch, S. Brain correlates of music-evoked emotions. *Nat. Rev. Neurosci.* **2014**, *15*, 170–180. [CrossRef]
24. Chen, S.-C.; Yeh, M.-L.; Chang, H.-J.; Lin, M.-F. Music, heart rate variability, and symptom clusters: A comparative study. *Support. Care Cancer* **2019**, *28*, 351–360. [CrossRef]
25. Pedersen, M.; Dam, C.; Rafaelsen, S. Music and pain during endorectal ultrasonography examination: A prospective questionnaire study and literature review. *Radiography* **2020**, *26*, e164–e169. [CrossRef] [PubMed]
26. Wren, A.A.; Shelby, R.A.; Soo, M.S.; Huysmans, Z.; Jarosz, J.A.; Keefe, F.J. Preliminary efficacy of a lovingkindness meditation intervention for patients undergoing biopsy and breast cancer surgery: A randomized controlled pilot study. *Support. Care Cancer* **2019**, *27*, 3583–3592. [CrossRef]
27. Bradt, J.; Dileo, C.; Myers-Coffman, K.; Biondo, J. Music interventions for improving psychological and physical outcomes in people with cancer. *Cochrane Database Syst. Rev.* **2021**, *2022*, CD006911. [CrossRef]
28. Choi, Y.K. The effect of music and progressive muscle relaxation on anxiety, fatigue, and quality of life in family caregivers of hospice patients. *J. Music. Ther.* **2010**, *47*, 53–69. [CrossRef] [PubMed]
29. Lai, H.-L.; Li, Y.-M.; Lee, L.-H. Effects of music intervention with nursing presence and recorded music on psycho-physiological indices of cancer patient caregivers. *J. Clin. Nurs.* **2011**, *21*, 745–756. [CrossRef] [PubMed]
30. Dingley, C.; Ruckdeschel, A.; Kotula, K.; Lekhak, N. Implementation and outcomes of complementary therapies in hospice care: An integrative review. *Palliat. Care Soc. Pract.* **2021**, *15*, 26323524211051753. [CrossRef]
31. Valero-Cantero, I.; Martínez-Valero, F.J.; Espinar-Toledo, M.; Casals, C.; Barón-López, F.J.; Vázquez, M. Complementary music therapy for cancer patients in at-home palliative care and their caregivers: Protocol for a multicentre randomised controlled trial. *BMC Palliat. Care* **2020**, *19*, 61. [CrossRef]
32. Valero-Cantero, I.; Casals, C.; Espinar-Toledo, M.; Barón-López, F.J.; Martínez-Valero, F.J.; Soler, N.G.-A.; Vázquez-Sánchez, M. Effect of Self-Chosen Music in Alleviating the Burden on Family Caregivers of Patients with Advanced Cancer: A Randomised Controlled Trial. *Int. J. Environ. Res. Public Health* **2023**, *20*, 4662. [CrossRef]
33. Ortiz, L.B.; González, G.M.C.; Chaparro-Diaz, L.; Herrera, B.S.; Rosero, E.V.; Carreño, S.P. Validez de constructo y confiabilidad del instrumento calidad de vida versión familiar en español. *Enfermería Glob.* **2015**, *14*, 227–249. [CrossRef]
34. Herdman, M.; Gudex, C.; Lloyd, A.; Janssen, M.; Kind, P.; Parkin, D.; Bonsel, G.; Badia, X. Development and preliminary testing of the new five-level version of EQ-5D (EQ-5D-5L). *Qual. Life Res.* **2011**, *20*, 1727–1736. [CrossRef]
35. Larsen, D.L.; Attkisson, C.; Hargreaves, W.A.; Nguyen, T.D. Assessment of client/patient satisfaction: Development of a general scale. *Eval. Program Plan.* **1979**, *2*, 197–207. [CrossRef] [PubMed]
36. Roberts, R.E.; Attkisson, C. Assessing client satisfaction among hispanics. *Evaluation Program Plan.* **1983**, *6*, 401–413. [CrossRef] [PubMed]
37. Hanser, S.B.; Butterfield-Whitcomb, J.; Kawata, M.; Collins, B.E. Home-based music strategies with individuals who have dementia and their family caregivers. *J. Music. Ther.* **2011**, *48*, 2–27. [CrossRef] [PubMed]
38. Butow, P.N.; The Australian Ovarian Cancer Study Group; Price, M.A.; Bell, M.L.; Webb, P.M.; Defazio, A.; Friedlander, M.; The Australian Ovarian Cancer Study Quality of Life Study Investigators. Caring for women with ovarian cancer in the last year of life: A longitudinal study of caregiver quality of life, distress and unmet needs. *Gynecol. Oncol.* **2014**, *132*, 690–697. [CrossRef]
39. Ito, E.; Tadaka, E. Effectiveness of the Online Daily Diary (ONDIARY) program on family caregivers of advanced cancer patients: A home-based palliative care trial. *Complement. Ther. Clin. Pract.* **2021**, *46*, 101508. [CrossRef]
40. Gabriel, I.; Creedy, D.; Coyne, E. Quality of life and associated factors among adults living with cancer and their family caregivers. *Nurs. Health Sci.* **2021**, *23*, 419–429. [CrossRef]
41. Ferrell, B.R.; Kravitz, K.; Borneman, T.; Friedmann, E.T. Family Caregivers: A Qualitative Study to Better Understand the Quality-of-Life Concerns and Needs of This Population. *Clin. J. Oncol. Nurs.* **2018**, *22*, 286–294. [CrossRef]
42. Gabriel, I.; Creedy, D.; Coyne, E. A systematic review of psychosocial interventions to improve quality of life of people with cancer and their family caregivers. *Nurs. Open* **2020**, *7*, 1299–1312. [CrossRef]
43. Kim, Y.; Carver, C.S. Unmet needs of family cancer caregivers predict quality of life in long-term cancer survivorship. *J. Cancer Surviv.* **2019**, *13*, 749–758. [CrossRef]
44. Chappell, N.L.; Reid, C. Burden and well-being among caregivers: Examining the distinction. *Gerontologist* **2002**, *42*, 772–780. [CrossRef]

45. Fu, F.; Zhao, H.; Tong, F.; Chi, I. A Systematic Review of Psychosocial Interventions to Cancer Caregivers. *Front. Psychol.* **2017**, *8*, 834. [CrossRef] [PubMed]
46. Batbaatar, E.; Dorjdagva, J.; Luvsannyam, A.; Savino, M.M.; Amenta, P. Determinants of patient satisfaction: A systematic review. *Perspect. Public Health* **2017**, *137*, 89–101. [CrossRef] [PubMed]

Disclaimer/Publisher's Note: The statements, opinions and data contained in all publications are solely those of the individual author(s) and contributor(s) and not of MDPI and/or the editor(s). MDPI and/or the editor(s) disclaim responsibility for any injury to people or property resulting from any ideas, methods, instructions or products referred to in the content.

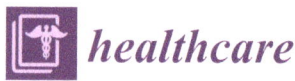

Review

Nursing Interventions in the Perioperative Pathway of the Patient with Breast Cancer: A Scoping Review

Mafalda Martins Cardoso [1,*], Cristina Lavareda Baixinho [1,2], Gilberto Tadeu Reis Silva [3] and Óscar Ferreira [1,2]

1. Nursing School of Lisbon, 1600-190 Lisbon, Portugal; crbaixinho@esel.pt (C.L.B.); oferreira@esel.pt (Ó.F.)
2. Nursing Research, Innovation and Development Centre of Lisbon (CIDNUR), 1900-160 Lisbon, Portugal
3. Stricto-Sensu Graduate Program at the School of Nursing, Federal University of Bahia, Salvador 40170-110, Brazil; gilberto.tadeu@ufba.br
* Correspondence: mcardoso@campus.esel.pt

Abstract: The decrease in average hospitalisation time and the increase in outpatient surgery in some types of breast cancer represent gains for the reduction of the negative impact of hospitalisation in women with breast cancer but are also a challenge for the organisation of nursing care to prepare women for surgery, reduce anxiety about the interventions, and ensure continuity of care in the postoperative period. The aim of this study is to identify nursing interventions present in the care provided to patients with breast cancer during the perioperative period. A scoping review was the method chosen to answer the research question: What are the specialised nursing interventions in the perioperative pathway of the patient with breast cancer? Inclusion and exclusion criteria were defined for the articles that were identified in the CINAHL and MEDLINE databases; later, additional sources were identified from the list of bibliographic references for each selected study. The final bibliographical sample consisted of seven articles, which allowed the identification of three key moments of nursing interventions in the perioperative period of patients with breast cancer: the preoperative consultation, the reception of the patient in the operating room, and the postoperative consultation. Factors such as psychological, emotional, and spiritual support, communication and patient-centred care, health education and surgical safety, and the definition of a perioperative pathway for these patients contribute significantly to patients' satisfaction and the improvement of their quality of life. The results of this study make it possible to establish recommendations for practise and for research, increasing the range of nurses' actions.

Keywords: cancer patient; breast cancer; nursing interventions; perioperative care; perioperative nursing consultation

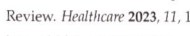

Citation: Cardoso, M.M.; Baixinho, C.L.; Silva, G.T.R.; Ferreira, Ó. Nursing Interventions in the Perioperative Pathway of the Patient with Breast Cancer: A Scoping Review. *Healthcare* **2023**, *11*, 1717. https://doi.org/10.3390/healthcare11121717

Academic Editor: Qiuping Li

Received: 28 April 2023
Revised: 8 June 2023
Accepted: 9 June 2023
Published: 12 June 2023

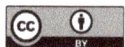

Copyright: © 2023 by the authors. Licensee MDPI, Basel, Switzerland. This article is an open access article distributed under the terms and conditions of the Creative Commons Attribution (CC BY) license (https://creativecommons.org/licenses/by/4.0/).

1. Introduction

Cancer is the second leading cause of death worldwide, and it is the second leading cause of death in Portugal [1]. The impact of this disease is not only felt by the patient but also represents an emotional and economic burden for the family and for society [2]. Breast cancer, specifically, is the most commonly diagnosed type of cancer and the second leading cause of death in women in Portugal [3]. The existence of population-based screenings with defined regularity that allow the diagnosis of pre-malignant lesions in their early stages leads to an increase in positive prognoses and a decrease in the mortality rate due to breast cancer. The most common therapeutic approach is surgery, sometimes associated with neoadjuvant or adjuvant treatments depending on the type and aggressivelness of the disease [4].

The therapeutic pathway of the patient with breast cancer consists of different stages, with the perioperative period being one of the treatment phases that implies a great effort on the part of the patient and her family and requires a good support network, a supportive health team, and comprehensive access to the health care system and community resources [5].

According to the Portuguese Association of Operating Room Nurses (AESOP), the perioperative period is the entirety of the preoperative, intraoperative, and postoperative moments, and perioperative care is a series of activities developed by perioperative nurses that tend to respond to the needs of the patient undergoing surgery and/or any invasive procedure [6].

Health professionals involved in the treatment of these patients must be aware of their pathway, demonstrating knowledge of the technical and scientific basis for the therapeutic options, thus contributing to a better adjustment of this person to their health/disease process. This knowledge also allows nurses to positively collaborate in the reorganisation of care, of information, and of the pathway itself through their active participation in institutional dynamics [7].

A study that aimed to examine under what conditions a patient might feel adequately prepared to go home and thereby be less likely to rate their length of stay as too short observed that one challenge in allowing patients to feel sufficiently informed and ready to go home is the reduced time for face-to-face consultations [8].

International recommendations advocate that all people proposed for surgery may have prehabilitation, right from the moment of the identified need for surgery, which enables the physical and psychological assessment of the person with the aim of creating a reference profile of the person's functional state, allowing the identification of deficits that can be solved or attenuated, preventing future complications [9]. The objectives of this process are to increase exercise capacity, increase muscular mass, improve nutritional status, and prepare the psychological condition [10,11].

Studies prove that the implementation of these programmes should start as soon as the person is proposed for surgery; however, for there to be results with the interventions implemented, the programme should last for 4 weeks [9–11].

A study that aimed to assess the feasibility and acceptability of an individualised, home-based prehabilitation intervention prior to breast cancer surgery and to explore the potential benefit of prehabilitation on physical fitness and participant-reported physical and psychosocial well-being over time observed that these may facilitate postoperative recovery, impact health behaviour change in the preoperative and postoperative periods, and improve physical activity levels and functional capacity both preoperatively and postoperatively [11].

It is consensual that the adequate preparation of these women has benefits for the reduction of costs associated with treatments while simultaneously keeping an important source of patients' satisfaction constant [6–8].

Based on the arguments mentioned above, the aim of this study is to identify nursing interventions in the care pathway of patients with breast cancer through their perioperative period.

2. Materials and Methods

2.1. Study Design

According to the aim of this study and due to the exploratory research carried out on the subject, it was considered that the scoping review was the appropriate method for this study as it constitutes "an ideal tool to determine the scope or coverage of a body of literature on a given topic and give a clear indication of the volume of literature and studies available as well as an overview (broad or detailed) of its focus" [12].

The protocol followed the six steps recommended for this type of systematic review: (1) identification of the review question; (2) designation of inclusion and exclusion criteria for studies and identification of relevant studies; (3) selection of studies to be included; (4) assessment of the level of evidence of the collected literature according to the JBI guidelines; (5) discussion of the results; and (6) synthesis and presentation of the obtained results [12–14].

Based on the question, "What nursing interventions are described in the literature as relevant in the care pathway of patients with breast cancer, through their perioperative period?" It was possible to define the eligibility criteria and the research strategy, with the perioperative period established as preoperative, intraoperative, and postoperative moments, more specifically during the preoperative consultation, the reception to the operating room, and the postoperative consultation. The concern with these 3 moments is due to the fact that, tendentially, an increasingly larger segment of surgeries is performed on an outpatient regimen or with a clear reduction in hospitalisation time, which implies a (re)organisation of care in order to monitor and intervene alongside these women through all these key moments of nursing contact.

2.2. Eligibility Criteria

The use of the acronym PCC (population, concept, and context) allowed the development of the previously presented research question. Each element of the acronym guided the definition of each specific inclusion criteria, presented in Table 1.

Table 1. Eligibility criteria according to the PCC acronym. Lisbon, 2022.

PCC	Inclusion Criteria	Exclusion Criteria
P	Adult female ($\geq$19 years) with breast cancer	Teenagers
C	Nursing interventions provided to the patient with breast cancer in the preoperative consultation, in the reception to the operating room, and in the postoperative consultation.	Inpatient nursing interventions. Nursing interventions in late postoperative period
C	Preoperative consultation, reception of the patient in the operating room, and postoperative consultation	Primary health care. Nursing homes. Rehabilitation units.

2.3. Data Collection

The research was carried out using the EBSCOhost database aggregator platform, specifically the CINAHL and MEDLINE databases, in November 2022. The search terms used were breast neoplasms, patients, patient-centred care, nursing interventions, perioperative care, and perioperative period, terms originally retrieved from the Health Sciences Descriptors site and indexed in each of the databases used. The Boolean operators OR and AND were used to operationalize the search, and language filters were applied for full text in Portuguese or English, excluding articles prior to 2017.

Table 2 presents the strategy used in the Medline database.

The search strategy included the use of 'natural' and indexed language. In CINHAL's search strategy, mesh is replaced by subject headings.

The screening of articles by title, abstract, and full article reading was carried out by two independent reviewers; a third element was activated in situations of non-consensus or doubt.

In a second phase, additional sources were identified from the list of bibliographical references for each selected study. A search was also carried out on Google Scholar and open-access scientific repositories using keywords and indexing terms.

2.4. Data Processing and Analysis

The researchers built an Excel table, shared in the cloud, to record the content extracted from the articles in the final bibliographic sample: identification of the title of the article/work; author(s), year of publication; type of article; objective(s), method, and main results/conclusions.

The articles that answered the research question and respected the inclusion criteria were subject to analysis, and a narrative synthesis of the results was carried out.

Table 2. Medline search strategy. Lisbon, 2022.

	Search Strategy	Number Articles
#1	((((((((((((((adult[Title/Abstract])) OR (elderly[Title/Abstract]))) OR (older person[Title/Abstract])) OR (older people[Title/Abstract]))) OR (age[Title/Abstract]))) OR (aged[Title/Abstract])) OR (elder*[Title/Abstract]))) OR (adult[MeSH Terms])) OR (aged[MeSH Terms])) OR (frail older adult[MeSH Terms]))) AND (woman[Title/Abstract])) NOT (adolescent[Title/Abstract]) Filters: Free full text, from 2017–2022	21,448
#2	((breast cancer[Title/Abstract])) OR (breast cancer[MeSH Terms]) Filters: Free full text, from 2017–2022	76,142
#3	(((((((((((((((nursing[Title/Abstract])) OR (nurs*[Title/Abstract])) OR (interv*[Title/Abstract])) OR (advanced Nurs*[Title/Abstract])) OR (educacional interventions[Title/Abstract])) OR (educat*[Title/Abstract])) OR (capacit*[Title/Abstract])) OR (nursing support[Title/Abstract])) OR (surgical nursing[Title/Abstract])) OR (advanced Nurs*[Title/Abstract])) OR (humanization[Title/Abstract])) OR (advanced practice nursing[MeSH Terms])) OR (early intervention[MeSH Terms])) OR (activities, educational[MeSH Terms])) OR (building, capacity[MeSH Terms])) Filters: Free full text, from 2017–2022	875,933
#4	((((((((((((consultation[Title/Abstract]) OR (consult*[Title/Abstract])) OR (preoperative consult*[Title/Abstract])) OR (postoperative consult*[Title/Abstract])) OR (admission to the operating room[Title/Abstract])) OR (operating room[Title/Abstract])) OR (ambulatory surgery[Title/Abstract])) OR (operating room[Title/Abstract])) OR (operating theater[Title/Abstract])) OR (care, postoperative[MeSH Terms])) OR (care, preoperative[MeSH Terms])) OR (period, preoperative[MeSH Terms])) OR (ambulatory surgery[MeSH Terms])) OR (ambulatory care facilities, hospital[MeSH Terms])Filters: Free full text, from 2017–2022	44,718
#5	#1 AND #2 AND #3 AND #4	5

3. Results

Figure 1 shows the PRISMA flowchart that describes the selection process, starting with 23 articles that were initially identified by applying the search terms in the databases, all of them from the CINAHL base, and 20 articles from searches performed on platforms such as Google Scholar and the Epistemonikos website. The final sample was comprised of seven articles that met the eligibility criteria and answered the research question.

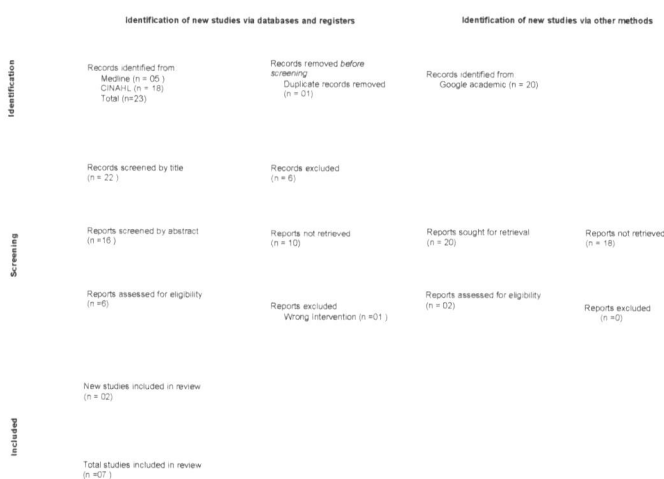

Figure 1. PRISMA-ScR flowchart. Lisbon, 2022.

Below, Table 3 shows the studies that comprise the final bibliographic sample [15–21].

Two systematic reviews of literature were identified [15,21]: a qualitative study [18], a methodological study [20]; a mixed descriptive study [16]; a correlational predictive study [19]; and a quasi-experimental study [17].

Of the seven selected studies, two refer to the Brazilian population [18,20]; one focuses on the Australian population [16]; another on Iranian women [19]; another on the Turkish population [17]; one in the US [15]; and one in Nigeria [21].

The content analysis of the included articles enabled the narrative synthesis that was organised according to the objectives into 3 points: nursing interventions throughout the preoperative consultation; nursing interventions during the patient's reception in the operating room; and nursing interventions throughout the postoperative consultation.

3.1. Nursing Interventions throughout the Preoperative Consultation

Regarding this perioperative moment, the interventions suggested in the selected articles refer specifically to aspects considered throughout the preoperative nursing consultation, focusing on knowledge about this stage of the breast cancer treatment, offering understanding for the person's situation, revealing an empathetic attitude, and providing psychological support. It is given great relevance to practical aspects of the preoperative preparation, such as the choice of a supportive bra, options related to breast implants, and the availability of support groups [16]. These aspects are reinforced by one other article [18], which points to the importance of attentive listening as a characteristic of communication with these patients and recommends a humanistic attitude, defined by emotional support and respect for the person's spirituality. This article also informs readers about the relevance of providing information about the perioperative pathway and the clarification of doubts related to surgical safety, such as regular medication or surgical preparation. It also advises the elaboration of guides or other informative strategies concerning the perioperative pathway, aiming to support patient education on the matter of preparing them for surgery and recovery.

Table 3. Final bibliographic sample. Lisbon, 2022.

Study/Country/Year	Study Design and Aim	Results
Wilson [15]. USA (2017)	Systematic review of literature. To describe how mobilization stretches and exercise decrease shoulder impairments, a complication related to breast cancer surgery, thus improving quality of life.	Prevent lymphedema. Observe patient's posture. Measure the circumference of both arms. Assess shoulder range. Measure BMI. Check exercise habits: type of exercise, duration, frequency, and intensity. Educate for exercise in the postoperative period. Reinforce the information about the exercises. Clarify doubts
Brown, Refeld, and Cooper [16]. Australia (2018)	Mixed descriptive study. To understand what, if any, differences exist in the perception of a breast care nurse (BCN) consultation between women who experienced a preoperative, face-to-face counselling and education opportunity with a BCN and those who required a telephone consultation or were unable to experience a preoperative BCN consultation.	Offer knowledge and understanding; Psychological support, empathy; Help with practical questions, information about breast implants, supportive bras, and support groups.
Nemli & Kartin [17]. Turkey (2019)	Quasi-experimental study. To determine the effects of exercise training that was supported with follow-up calls at home on the postoperative level of physical activity and quality of life of women with breast cancer.	Measurement of the upper limbs; Training of the exercises available in the brochure, clarifying doubts; Reinforce the importance of exercise and clarify doubts;
Trescher, et al. [18]. Brazil (2019)	Qualitative study. To know the care needs in the preoperative period for tumour resection in the perception of women with breast cancer and nurses	Attentive listening; emotional support. Transmission of information about the patient's pathway, clarification of doubts about therapy, and surgical preparation. Design guides and strategies for providing patient orientation. Understanding the spiritual dimension and its place in the treatment of the person.
Ghaffari, et al. [19]. Iran (2020)	Correlational predictive study. To determine the predictive values of patient-centred communication (PCC) and patient characteristics on body image (BI) perception in postmastectomy patients.	Build a trusting relationship; Enhance the patient's involvement in decision-making; Information exchange; Respond to emotional needs; Help manage uncertainty; Support the patient's independence by providing appropriate resources.

Table 3. Cont.

Study/Country/Year	Study Design and Aim	Results
Trescher, et al. Brazil [20]. (2020)	Methodological study Development of a model for nursing consultation in the preoperative period of women with breast cancer at an oncological outpatient.	List of nursing interventions according to the NANDA-I taxonomy; Planned activities; Expected results
Tola, Chow, and Liang [21]. Nigeira (2021)	Systematic review of literature To identify, analyse, and synthesise the effects of non-pharmacological interventions on preoperative anxiety and acute postoperative pain in women undergoing breast cancer surgery.	Use of music therapy to reduce pre- and postoperative anxiety; Postoperative aromatherapy in pain management; Acupuncture to reduce anxiety and pain.

Two articles [15,17] focus on the prevention of complications associated with immobility, recommending the preoperative assessment of the patients' physical condition, the evaluation of body mass index (BMI), an examination of their posture and range of mobility of the upper limbs, and the documentation of the patient's routine physical activity. They emphasise the importance of the nurses' role in education about the benefits of exercise and prehabilitation while preparing for surgery and as agents for motivation and self-efficacy, all important factors promoting recovery in the postoperative period. Both articles aim to prevent complications such as lymphedema and improve the quality of life of these patients.

One article discusses a model of person-centred communication as a fundamental tool for creating a relationship of trust, guaranteeing spiritual and psychological support, promoting the engagement of patients in the decision-making processes, and conducing to better outcomes when confronted with self-image problems [19].

Lastly, one article provides a list of nursing interventions, resorting to the NANDA-I taxonomy (International's Nursing Diagnosis), allowing us to confer the activities planned for each nursing intervention as well as the results that can be expected [20].

3.2. Nursing Interventions during the Patient's Reception in the Operating Room

Of the totality of the articles selected for this review, only one makes a brief reference to the moment of the patient's reception in the operating room and the importance of nursing interventions during this transition of care [21]. The article consists of a systematic review of the literature on the effects of non-pharmacological interventions in the reduction of preoperative anxiety, referring to an article [22] that reports on the impact of music therapy in the reduction of anxiety when used during the patient's transference to the operating room.

3.3. Nursing Interventions troughout the Postoperative Consultation

Regarding the postoperative consultation moment, the selected articles inform about the importance of the nurse's role in meeting the emotional and physical needs of the patients [16]. Two studies [15,17] refer to the follow-up consultation after breast surgery with the purpose of promoting physical exercise and preventing the risks of immobility and the formation of lymphedema, demonstrating positive results in improving the quality of life of patients who comply with the recommended exercise schemes.

The article dedicated to person-centred communication [19] focuses on the impact of this style of communication on the self-image perception of women undergoing mastectomy, revealing benefits linked to patient empowerment and stating the importance of training nurses in this type of communication.

One article reveals that music therapy and acupuncture are significant resources for controlling postoperative pain in patients undergoing breast surgery [21].

4. Discussion

This scoping review allowed the mapping of nursing interventions in the perioperative period of patients with breast cancer, identifying the main nursing interventions throughout preoperative and postoperative nursing consultations as well as during the reception to the operating room.

In this regard, the nursing interventions here identified should be added to those already existing in preoperative consultation protocols, namely the importance given to the prevention of postoperative lymphedema in women undergoing axillary dissection, such as the assessment of the physical state, physical activity, and the perimeters of the upper limbs, and the training of exercises recommended for the first phase of the postoperative period [15,17]. These interventions must subsequently be reassessed and reinforced in the postoperative consultation, documented in the patient's clinical file, and made available to the other members of the health team to ensure continuity of care [20].

The emphasis on physical exercise as a rehabilitation mechanism needs to be prioritised and schooled, not only among patients but also among health professionals, so that it can be included and considered relevant for patients' education, allowing it to reveal an effective impact on motivation and a change in behaviours [23,24].

In general, the reduction of anxiety seems to be one of the main objectives of nursing interventions in the perioperative period, contributing in a valuable way to patients' satisfaction with the care provided and to a more positive perception of well-being [18,21–23]. A wide variety of approaches aiming to reduce anxiety have recently been recommended for the perioperative context, including education and training in relaxation techniques, deep breathing exercises, meditation, yoga, and music therapy [25].

Psychological and emotional support are also widely mentioned in the selected articles, formulating nursing interventions to be considered in all approaches to patients and, in particular, to patients with breast cancer, taking into account the impact of the surgery on these women's lives and self-image as a cause of disruption in the person's self-concept as a woman, mother, or wife in both social and professional contexts [19]. The involvement of the family in the context of care is also one of the needs expressed by women, family members, and caregivers who must be included in the care plan [26].

While attending to the patient, it is essential to ensure the cooperation of a cohesive and communicative multidisciplinary team that shares relevant information to guarantee an effective and satisfactory pathway for the patient, the family, and the health team. From the patients' point of view, there are several benefits to this interprofessional collaboration in order to promote the success of the treatments, since effective teamwork tends to increase patient satisfaction, improve access to health care, and favour health outcomes [27].

In the perioperative context, it is essential to have a preoperative nursing consultation aimed at women with breast cancer, oriented towards the main differences in the staging and treatment options, with knowledge of the main complications and the skills to identify the desired health outcomes; to be able to welcome the patient to the operating room in a humanised and personal environment, meeting the emotional, psychological, and spiritual needs of this person; and to hold a post-operative consultation sensitive to the pathway travelled, aiming for the satisfaction of the patient and her family, the reduction of their anxiety, and efficiently identifying and promptly resolving problems. Preoperative health education, accomplished through nursing consultations (in person or over the phone), focusing on the patient, adjusting the nurse's attention to the patient's individual needs, promoting bidirectional communication, encouraging shared decision-making, and ensuring adequate training of nurses in communication skills and techniques are some of the key factors for optimising perioperative practises [28].

Wu et al. [29] investigated to determine the feasibility of multimodal prehabilitation as part of the breast cancer treatment pathway, and the results of the pilot study showed that patients would overwhelmingly like to participate in this programme (81.3%) as part of their breast cancer treatment and that the programme is feasible and can be delivered.

The results of a recent systematic review reinforce the potential of prehabilitation in the preoperative preparation of women with breast cancer to optimise clinical, physical, and psychological outcomes; however, the authors are aware that researchers and healthcare professionals need to have more knowledge about the effects of unimodal and multimodal interventions implemented in the preoperative period and their effects [30].

The existence of a single study that explores the reception of women in the operating room stands out in this review. Future studies should explore the importance of this activity since studies inform us that a structured reception helps to reduce patients' anxiety, clarify doubts, prepare the discharge process, guarantee continuity of care, and manage expectations regarding the disease and self-care when returning home [21,22,31,32].

The limitations of this review are due to some methodological options, such as restrictions placed on the language and free access to full text, which allowed some articles to be excluded deductively that may have respected the inclusion criteria. It should also be noted that the studies are heterogeneous, and it was decided not to assess their methodological quality.

5. Conclusions

The results obtained in this review contribute to the enrichment of knowledge concerning the needs expressed by women with breast cancer in their surgical pathway and also inform about some of the nursing interventions that must be considered throughout the perioperative period.

The information collected in this scoping review completes the knowledge that perioperative nurses already possess on the prevention of surgical risks, increasing the scope of action of these professionals and connecting them to other hospital structures involved in the treatment of these patients, such as in-patient services or specialty consultations such as breast and oncology consultations. Thereby, the role of the specialist nurse in oncology nursing proves to be of great importance in the training of teams and in the identification of the most appropriate interventions for each case on an individual basis.

From the research point of view, it is suggested that the design and evaluation of nursing interventions be done for each of the three moments described: preoperative consultation, reception in the operating room, and postoperative consultation, given that the research did not allow the identification of structured and rigorously evaluated programmes that allow evidence-based recommendations.

Author Contributions: Conceptualization, M.M.C. and Ó.F.; methodology, M.M.C., C.L.B., Ó.F. and G.T.R.S.; software, M.M.C., Ó.F. and G.T.R.S.; validation, C.L.B. and Ó.F.; formal analysis, M.M.C., Ó.F., C.L.B. and G.T.R.S.; investigation, M.M.C., C.L.B. and Ó.F.; resources, C.L.B. and Ó.F.; data curation, M.M.C., C.L.B. and Ó.F.; writing—original draft preparation, M.M.C., C.L.B. and Ó.F.; writing—review and editing, M.M.C., C.L.B., Ó.F. and G.T.R.S.; supervision, Ó.F. project administration, M.M.C.; funding acquisition, C.L.B. and Ó.F. All authors have read and agreed to the published version of the manuscript.

Funding: The present study was funded by the Centre for Research, Innovation, and Development in Nursing in Portugal by means of grants provided to some of the authors (CIDNUR, Psafe2transition_2021).

Institutional Review Board Statement: Not applicable.

Informed Consent Statement: Not applicable.

Data Availability Statement: Data are available only upon request to the authors.

Conflicts of Interest: The authors declare no conflict of interest.

References

1. Direção Geral da Saúde. *Programa Nacional para as Doenças Oncológicas—Recursos do SNS em Oncologia—Relatório de Inquérito*; Direção Geral da Saúde: Lisbon, Portugal, 2020.
2. Direção Geral da Saúde. *Programa Nacional para as Doenças Oncológicas*; Direção Geral da Saúde: Lisbon, Portugal, 2017.
3. World Health Organization. International Agency for Researcher on Cancer. *Cancer Today* **2022**. Available online: https://gco.iarc.fr/today/online-analysis-table?v=2020&mode=cancer&mode_population=continents&population=900&populations=620&key=asr&sex=2&cancer=39&type=0&statistic=5&prevalence=0&population_group=0&ages_group%5B%5D=0&ages_group%5B%5D=17&group_cancer=1&i (accessed on 22 February 2023).
4. Alves, R.S.; Bártolo, J. Tratamento cirúrgico do carcinoma da mama. In *Manual de Oncologia SPO: Abordagem e Tratamento do Cancro da Mama*; Sociedade de Portuguesa de Oncologia: Lisbon, Portugal, 2020; pp. 107–126.
5. Seiler, A.; Jenewein, J. Resilience in cancer patients. *Front. Psychiatry* **2019**, *10*, 208. [CrossRef] [PubMed]
6. Associação dos Enfermeiros de Sala de Operações Portugueses. *Enfermagem Perioperatória: Da Filosofia à Prática de Cuidados*; Lusodidacta: Loures, Portugal, 2006.
7. Kaptain, K.; Ulsøe, M.; Dreyer, P. Surgical perioperative pathways—Patient experiences of unmet needs show that a person-centred approach is needed. *J. Clin. Nurs.* **2019**, *28*, 2214–2224. [CrossRef] [PubMed]
8. Nowak, M.; Lee, S.; Karbach, U.; Pfaff, H.; Groß, S.E. Short length of stay and the discharge process: Preparing breast cancer patients appropriately. *Patient Educ. Couns.* **2019**, *102*, 2318–2324. [CrossRef] [PubMed]
9. Carli, F.; Gillis, C.; Scheede-Bergdahl, C. Promoting a culture of prehabilitation for the surgical cancer patient. *Acta Oncol.* **2017**, *56*, 128–133. [CrossRef]
10. Boudreaux, A.; Simmons, J. Prehabilitation and Optimization of Modifiable Patient Risk Factors: The Importance of Effective Preoperative Evaluation to Improve Surgical Outcomes. *AORN J.* **2019**, *109*, 500–507. [CrossRef]
11. Brahmbhatt, P.; Sabiston, C.M.; Lopez, C.; Chang, E.; Goodman, J.; Jones, J.; McCready, D.; Randall, I.; Rotstein, S.; Santa Mina, D. Feasibility of Prehabilitation Prior to Breast Cancer Surgery: A Mixed-Methods Study. *Front. Oncol.* **2020**, *10*, 571091. [CrossRef]
12. Munn, Z.; Peters, M.D.J.; Stern, C.; Tufanaru, C.; McArthur, A.; Aromataris, E. Systematic review or scoping review? Guidance for authors when choosing between a systematic or scoping review approach. *BMC Med. Res. Methodol.* **2018**, *18*, 143. [CrossRef]
13. Peters, M.D.; Marnie, C.; Tricco, A.C.; Pollock, D.; Munn, Z.; Alexander, L.; McInerney, P.; Godfrey, C.M.; Khalil, H. Updated methodological guidance for the conduct of scoping reviews. *JBI Evid. Synth.* **2020**, *18*, 2119–2126. [CrossRef]
14. Tricco, A.C.; Lillie, E.; Zarin, W.; O'Brien, K.K.; Colquhoun, H.; Levac, D.; Moher, D.; Peters, M.D.J.; Horsley, T.; Weeks, L.; et al. PRISMA extension for scoping reviews (PRISMA-ScR): Checklist and explanation. *Ann. Intern. Med.* **2018**, *169*, 467–473. [CrossRef]
15. Wilson, D.J. Exercise for the patient after breast cancer surgery. *Semin. Oncol. Nurs.* **2017**, *33*, 98–105. [CrossRef]
16. Brown, J.; Refeld, G.; Cooper, A. Timing and mode of breast care nurse consultation from the patient's perspective. *Oncol. Nurs. Forum* **2018**, *45*, 389–398. [CrossRef]
17. Nemli, A.; Kartin, P.T. Effects of exercise training and follow-up calls at home on physical activity and quality of life after a mastectomy. *Jpn. J. Nurs. Sci.* **2019**, *16*, 322–328. [CrossRef] [PubMed]
18. Trescher, G.P.; Amante, L.N.; Rosa, L.M.; Balbinot Reis Girondi, J.; Severo Varela, A.I.; Oro, J.; Mancia Rolim, J.; dos Santos, M.J. Needs of women with breast cancer in the pre-operative period. *J. Nurs.* **2019**, *13*, 1288–1294. [CrossRef]
19. Ghaffari, F.; Ghahramanian, A.; Zamanzadeh, V.; Onyeka, T.C.; Davoodi, A.; Mazaheri, E.; Asghari-Jafarabadi, M. Patient-centred communication for women with breast cancer: Relation to body image perception. *J. Clin. Nurs.* **2020**, *29*, 4674–4684. [CrossRef] [PubMed]
20. Trescher, G.P.; Amante, L.N.; Da Rosa, L.M.; Girondi, J.B.R.; Miranda, G.M.; Santos, M.J.D.; Zuanazzi, E.C.; Mohr, H.S.S. Sistematização da consulta de enfermagem em pré-operatório às mulheres com câncer de mama. *Enferm. Foco* **2020**, *11*, 40–47. Available online: http://revista.cofen.gov.br/index.php/enfermagem/article/view/3400/1022 (accessed on 23 May 2023).
21. Tola, Y.O.; Chow, K.M.; Liang, W. Effects of non-pharmacological interventions on preoperative anxiety and postoperative pain in patients undergoing breast cancer surgery: A systematic review. *J. Clin. Nurs.* **2021**, *30*, 3369–3384. [CrossRef]
22. Palmer, J.B.; Lane, D.; Mayo, D.; Schluchter, M.; Leeming, R. Effects of music therapy on anesthesia requirements and anxiety in women undergoing ambulatory breast surgery for cancer diagnosis and treatment: A randomized controlled trial. *J. Clin. Oncol.* **2015**, *33*, 3162–3168. [CrossRef]
23. Gonçalves, M.A.; Cerejo, M.N.; Martins, J.C. The influence of the information provided by nurses on preoperative anxiety. *RER* **2017**, *IV*, 17–29. [CrossRef]
24. Yeon, S.; Jeong, A.; Min, J.; Byeon, J.; Yoon, Y.J.; Heo, J.; Lee, C.; Kim, J.; Park, S.; Kim, S.I.; et al. Tearing down the barriers to exercise after mastectomy: A qualitative inquiry to facilitate exercise among breast cancer survivors. *BMJ Open* **2022**, *12*, e055157. [CrossRef]
25. Carli, F.; Silver, J.K.; Feldman, L.S.; McKee, A.; Gilman, S.; Gillis, C.; Scheede-Bergdahl, C.; Gamsa, A.; Stout, N.; Hirsch, B. Surgical prehabilitation in patients with cancer: State-of-the-science and recommendations for future research from a panel of subject matter experts. *Phys. Med. Rehabil. Clin. N. Am.* **2017**, *28*, 49–64. [CrossRef]
26. Fuentes-Ramírez, A.; Laverde-Contreras, O.L. Nursing intervention to meet the family members' needs during the surgery waiting time. *Rev. Lat. Am. Enferm.* **2021**, *29*, e3483. [CrossRef]

27. Kurniasih, D.A.A.; Setiawati, E.P.; Pradipta, I.S.; Subarnas, A. Patients' Perspectives of Interprofessional Collaboration in Breast Cancer Unit. *Healthcare* **2023**, *11*, 332. [CrossRef] [PubMed]
28. Fernández Fernández, E.; Fernández-Ordoñez, E.; García-Gamez, M.; Guerra-Marmolejo, C.; Iglesias-Parra, R.; Soler, N.G.; González-Cano-Caballero, M. Indicators and predictors modifiable by the nursing department during the preoperative period: A scoping review. *J. Clin. Nurs.* **2023**, *32*, 2339–2360. [CrossRef] [PubMed]
29. Wu, F.; Laza-Cagigas, R.; Pagarkar, A.; Olaoke, A.; El Gammal, M.; Rampal, T. The Feasibility of Prehabilitation as Part of the Breast Cancer Treatment Pathway. *PM&R* **2021**, *13*, 1237–1246. [CrossRef]
30. Toohey, K.; Hunter, M.; McKinnon, K.; Casey, T.; Turner, M.; Taylor, S.; Paterson, C. A systematic review of multimodal prehabilitation in breast cancer. *Breast Cancer Res. Treat.* **2023**, *197*, 1–37. [CrossRef] [PubMed]
31. Kennedy, E.D.; McKenzie, M.; Schmocker, S.; Jeffs, L.; Cusimano, M.D.; Pooni, A.; Nenshi, R.; Scheer, A.S.; Forbes, T.L.; McLeod, R.S. Patient engagement study to identify and improve surgical experience. *Br. J. Surg.* **2021**, *108*, 435–440. [CrossRef] [PubMed]
32. Cruz, C.S.R.; Baixinho, C.L.; Bernardes, R.A.; Ferreira, Ó.R. Nursing Interventions for Head and Neck Cancer Patients That Promote Embracement in the Operating Room/Surgery Unit: A Near-Empty Scoping Review. *Nurs. Rep.* **2022**, *12*, 912–921. [CrossRef]

Disclaimer/Publisher's Note: The statements, opinions and data contained in all publications are solely those of the individual author(s) and contributor(s) and not of MDPI and/or the editor(s). MDPI and/or the editor(s) disclaim responsibility for any injury to people or property resulting from any ideas, methods, instructions or products referred to in the content.

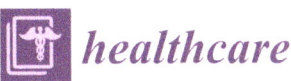

Review

Foot Health in People with Cancer Undergoing Chemotherapy: A Scoping Review

Raquel Veiga-Seijo [1,2,3,*] and Cristina Gonzalez-Martin [1,2,3]

1. Department of Health Sciences, Faculty of Nursing and Podiatry, Campus Esteiro, Campus Industrial de Ferrol, Universidade da Coruña, 15471 Ferrol, Spain; cristina.gmartin@udc.es
2. Research Group in Nursing and Health Care, Instituto de Investigación Biomédica de A Coruña (INIBIC), Hospital Universitario de A Coruña (HUAC), Universidade da Coruña, Sergas, 15006 A Coruña, Spain
3. Research Group in Rheumatology and Health (GIR-S), Faculty of Physiotherapy, Campus Oza, Universidade da Coruña, 15008 A Coruña, Spain
* Correspondence: raquel.veiga.seijo@udc.es

Abstract: Background: Chemotherapy has relevant implications for cancer patients' physical, social, and psychological health. Foot health has gained relevance in recent years due to its importance to independence and wellbeing, especially in chronic conditions. This study aims to explore the scope of the literature regarding foot health problems in people with cancer undergoing chemotherapy. Methods: scoping review following the PRISMA-ScR, Arksey and O'Malley, and the Joanna Briggs Institute guidelines. Different databases were used (Cochrane Plus, Scopus, Web of Science, and Pubmed). A total of 4911 articles were identified. Finally, 11 papers were included. Results: Foot problems are relevant and deteriorate wellbeing. The prevalence of some podiatric pathologies is controversial. The main literature deals with hand–foot syndrome and peripheral neuropathy. Focused instruments on foot health were not thoroughly used. Conclusion: There is insufficient evidence on foot health problems and their influence on the quality of life of people with cancer undergoing chemotherapy. Even though a significant percentage of this population has a foot problem, its care and importance are neglected. More studies are needed to contribute to the care of people with cancer through foot health.

Keywords: cancer; foot; quality of life; chemotherapy; scoping review; evidence-based practice; oncology; podiatry

1. Introduction

Cancer is a health condition with outstanding morbidity and mortality and is the second cause of death worldwide [1,2]. It presents an increasing trend worldwide, with an estimated 28.4 million cases in 2040 [3,4]. The relevance of this problem is shown in its magnitude and the implications that this health condition adds to the multidimensional complex of people's wellbeing.

The quality of life (QoL) of people with cancer is one of the most relevant concerns in the field of oncology [5] since cancer is the disease that causes the most significant loss of years of healthy life [6]. This is due to the consequences that adverse treatment events have on people's health, not only during treatment but also after it. Chemotherapy is one of the most common methods, and there is an increase in morbidity and mortality with the number of people requiring it [7]. Therefore, the development of adverse events seems to be an essential factor that contributes to the decrease in people's QoL [8,9].

Several studies were found in the literature on the adverse effects that chemotherapy treatments trigger. Specifically, research over the past two decades has highlighted adverse effects, such as skin and nail toxicity or peripheral neuropathy [8,9], and their implications for people's QoL. However, knowledge about these effects on foot health is invisible and neglected, despite the critical role that feet play in maintaining a healthy lifestyle [10,11]. In fact, only two articles refer to foot health [12,13].

At present, this gap in the literature is striking since other studies have shown the negative impact that podiatric problems have on general and health-related QoL, constituting a determinant of health [14]. In the field of oncology, this can also be very important, since people may feel limited in the way they face the disease process, in activities of daily living, in maintaining healthy lifestyle habits, and in having an active lifestyle within the possibilities during the oncological process.

In addition, the context described above is significantly different from the attention that other conditions have received in the scientific literature and in clinical practice in the field of foot health. In other health fields associated with chronic conditions [15], such as Diabetes Mellitus or Rheumatoid Arthritis, literature and implications for clinical practice are emerging in which foot problems are highly relevant, such as foot pain, structural alterations, and skin changes [16–18]. Likewise, today, the concern that amputations have for people with diabetes and health services is well known.

Taking into account the above context, the relevance and need to focus on foot health in this field are due to its role in posture and ambulation and its responsibility for autonomy, independence, and wellbeing [10]. In general, foot problems are known in the general population, and their identification is key since they have an impact on people's general health. People with cancer have complex and multidimensional circumstances, and the current agenda requires interdisciplinary healthcare professionals to contribute to their QoL. Given that podiatric adverse events may interfere with the general and podiatric wellbeing of people with cancer, it is pertinent to better understand the effects on foot health in people receiving chemotherapy.

Up to now, no review has been found that explores the published literature on foot health problems in people with cancer undergoing chemotherapy. Therefore, it is necessary to determine to what extent and how this issue has been described in the literature. This scoping review aims to explore the scope of the literature regarding foot health problems in people with cancer undergoing chemotherapy.

For this reason, this study is proposed to summarize the current scientific evidence on the topic addressed, to determine the relevance of future research and in which direction it should be oriented, as well as to provide new information for clinical practice.

2. Materials and Methods

A systematic review was carried out based on the "Scoping Review" methodology, following the guidelines of Arksey and O'Malley [19] and PRISMA-ScR [20]. The purpose is to be an initial point of investigation in the exposed field, evaluating the magnitude and scope of the existing literature. Levac et al. [21] and guidelines from the Joanna Brigss Institute [22] were followed to ensure methodological rigor. According to its theoretical framework, this scoping review includes five phases that are shown below.

2.1. Identifying the Research Question (Stage 1)

The research question formulated in this scoping review is as follows: What is known about the foot health problems of people with cancer undergoing chemotherapy?

2.2. Identifying Relevant Studies (Stage 2)

A search strategy was carried out that involved several phases, beginning with the identification of key search terms. For this purpose, the Participant, Concept, and Context (PCC) framework recommended by the Joanna Briggs Institute [22] was taken into account: P: people with cancer older than 18 years, C: foot health problems, and C: chemotherapy treatment for cancer. From this framework, a test search was carried out with an initial strategy that was consulted and supported by specialists in database formation from the university. The final search strategy was carried out in February 2022 and reviewed in December 2022. Table 1 shows the search terms.

Table 1. Search terms.

Concept	Search Terms
Foot	Foot OR podiatry OR "hand–foot syndrome" OR "foot diseases" OR "foot health"
Cancer	Neoplasm OR cancer
Chemotherapy	"Drug therapy" OR "chemotherapy"

In accordance with the referenced theoretical framework [19], to identify potentially relevant documents, different electronic databases related to Health Sciences were used: Cochrane Library Plus, Pubmed, Web of Science, and Scopus. All original articles, reviews, and conference papers published in Spanish, Portuguese, and English in the last 15 years were considered for inclusion. Search terms were applied to the title, abstract, and keyword fields. Only those publications that addressed foot health problems in adult people receiving chemotherapy were included.

2.3. Study Selection (Stage 3)

All the authors reviewed the publications obtained and discussed the results. First, the documents were identified according to the title and abstract. Most of the discarded articles addressed the effectiveness of cancer therapies and were partly analyzed based on the adverse effects they triggered. Among them, reference was made to hand–foot syndrome, but without addressing foot health or responding to the objective of this work. Another significant volume of discarded papers addressed pathophysiological aspects of chemotherapy-induced peripheral neuropathy. Subsequently, the full text was reviewed, resolving disagreements if they occurred.

2.4. Charting the Data (Stage 4)

At first, the documents were saved in Mendeley and arranged in a Microsoft Word table. Two researchers reviewed each article. They were organized by author, year and place of publication, study population, methodology, and main results.

2.5. Collecting, Summarizing, and Reporting the Results (Stage 5)

The analysis was performed using a descriptive analysis (including n and percentage) and a thematic analysis (Braun and Clarke [23]), following both inductive and deductive approaches.

3. Results

A total of 4911 articles were initially found. Finally, 11 articles fulfilled the previously established criteria (Figure 1). Table 2 shows the bibliometric and general characteristics of the studies analyzed, the foot health problems, and the foot health problems related to QoL in people with cancer undergoing chemotherapy.

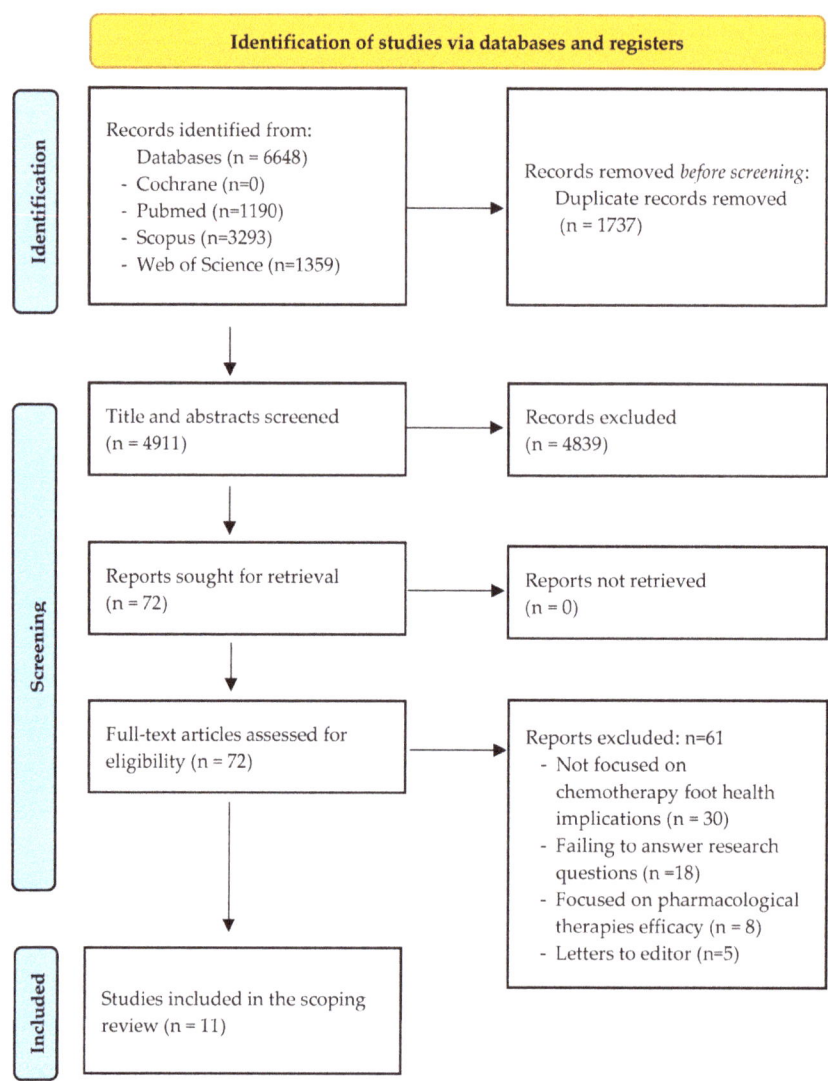

Figure 1. PRISMA flow diagram showing the studies included and excluded.

Table 2. Bibliometric characteristics, foot health problems, and foot health problems related to QoL in people with cancer undergoing chemotherapy [12,13,24-32].

First Author, Year, Country (Health Professional Department)	Journal	Sample	Anticancer Therapies	Type of Study	Research Objectives	Data Collection Methods Concerning Foot	Was the Aim of the Study the Foot Health?	Studied Foot Health Problems Related QoL	Main Findings
Lacouture et al. [13], 2018, USA (Department of Oncology and Podiatry)	Journal of the American Podiatric Medical Association	n = 291 Breast (40.2%), colon (10.3%)	Cytotoxic chemotherapy, targeted therapy, radiation therapy, surgical procedures, and stem cell transplants	Clinical experience and literature review	To show the impact of podiatric adverse events on QoL in an Oncology Foot Care Program and to review podiatric adverse events related to cancer treatments.	NCICTCAE	Yes	Yes	• *Foot health problems* • *Foot health problems related to Quality of Life (QoL)* • *Foot health problems* Podiatric adverse events from anticancer therapies are highlighted. The main problems are nail toxicities, hand–foot syndrome (HFS), edema, xerosis, hyperkeratosis, and neuropathy. • *Foot health problems related to QoL*. The adverse effects negatively impact people's QoL. Hence, it is important to prevent and manage podiatric adverse events because these effects may result in the interruption, diminution, or discontinuation of cancer treatments.
Komatsu et al. [24], 2019, Japan, Yagasaki, Hirata, and Hamamoto (Department of Nursing)	European Journal of Oncology Nursing	n = 20 (13 female, 7 male) colon (65%), gastric (20%) cancer	Chemotherapy and targeted therapy	Qualitative study	To understand the perceived needs of advanced-stage cancer patients with chemotherapy-related hand–foot syndrome and/or targeted therapy-related hand-foot skin reactions.	Interviews	Focused on HFS	Yes	• *Foot health problems* Participants experienced pain and a change in sensitivity, describing the feet as an integral part of mobility, which affects the activities of daily living. • *Foot health problems related to QoL*. Four themes emerged about the needs of people with chemotherapy-related HFS: a sense of helplessness with persistent symptoms, noticeable appearance as a barrier to social participation, decreased willingness to work and continue treatment, and the need for individual coping strategies. These unmet needs are not often voiced. Hence, health care providers must be involved in this problem.

Table 2. Cont.

First Author, Year, Country (Health Professional Department)	Journal	Sample	Anticancer Therapies	Type of Study	Research Objectives	Data Collection Methods Concerning Foot	Was the Aim of the Study the Foot Health?	Studied Foot Health Problems Related QoL	Main Findings
Hsu et al. [25], 2019, Taiwan (Department of Nursing)	European Journal of Oncology Nursing	n = 85 breast cancer (100% female)	Docetaxel-based chemotherapy	Cross-sectional, descriptive, and correlational designs	(1) to assess breast cancer patients' perceived levels of HFS-related foot symptoms, HFS-related hand or finger symptoms, and HFS-related restrictions in daily activities, and (2) to identify factors associated with HFS-related restrictions in daily activities.	Hand–Foot Quality of Life Scale (HF QoLS) symptom subscale questionnaire HF QoLS—daily activity subscale NCICTCAE	Focused on Hand–Foot Syndrome	Yes	• *Foot health problems* The foot stands out as the body part most affected in relation to HFS. Participants reported a higher level of HFS-related foot symptoms than in hands or fingers. They observed that 41.2% of people with breast cancer reported this effect. The symptoms presented a higher mean in the feet (8.76 ± 0.72) than in the hands (7.62 ± 0.70). • *Foot health problems related to QoL* The restriction in daily activities was associated more with foot symptoms, which explained 44.7% of the variance in the restriction of activities.
Miller et al. [32], 2014, USA (Department of Dermatology)	Journal of the American Academy of Dermatology	Breast cancer	Different chemotherapy agents and targeted multikinase inhibitors	Review	To describe the epidemiology, pathogenesis, clinical presentation, and current evidence-based treatment for chemotherapy-induced hand–foot syndrome and nail changes.	HFS: National Cancer Institute Criteria for its classification and World Health Organization criteria Nail: NCICTCAE	Focused on Hand–Foot Syndrome and nail changes (both hand and foot)	Yes	• *Foot health problems* HFS can affect palms, soles, dorsal hands, and feet, with erythema and edema accompanied by the onset of neuropathic pain. It can progress to blistering with desquamation, erosion, and ulceration. HFS was initially described as tingling and burning pain. Subsequently, the sensation of pain and temperature decrease, and neuropathic symptoms begin, accompanied by erythema and edema palmoplantar. Nail changes such as onycholisis, Beau lines, subungual hemorrhage, nail pigmentation, paronychia, and splinter hemorrhage can occur in up to 88% of patients. • *Foot health problems related to QoL* These problems may cause cosmetic concern, pain, infection, and an impact on QoL. They may involve reducing the dose of chemotherapy or even having to stop treatment and switch to another. They are common complications of many classic agents.

Table 2. Cont.

First Author, Year, Country (Health Professional Department)	Journal	Sample	Anticancer Therapies	Type of Study	Research Objectives	Data Collection Methods Concerning Foot	Was the Aim of the Study the Foot Health?	Studied Foot Health Problems Related QoL	Main Findings
Gilbar et al. [30], 2009, Australia (Department of Pharmacology)	Journal of Oncology Pharmacy Practice	Articles about breast, lung, ovarian, and colon cancer, melanoma, Hodgkin, and carcinoid tumors	Different chemotherapy agents	Literature Review	To provide a comprehensive literature review of chemotherapy-induced nail toxicity (presentation, implication, drugs, and approaches for prevention and management).	NCICTCAE	Focused on nails (both hand and foot)	No	• *Foot health problems* Nail toxicity is a relatively uncommon adverse effect. The clinical presentation varies depending on the chemotherapeutic agent, the nail structure affected, and the severity. Taxane and anthracyclines are the most prevalent drugs related to this toxicity. The most common nail problems were: Beau's lines, onychomadesis, Mees's lines, melanonychia, onycholysis, Muehrcke's lines, splinter hemorrhage, subungual hematoma, and paronychia. • *Foot health problems related to QoL* It may involve cosmetic concerns, pain, discomfort, and negative implications for QoL and DLA. It is necessary to develop a healthcare program about the potential nail toxicities.
Palomo-López et al. [12], 2017, Spain (Department of Nursing and Podiatry)	Cancer Management and Research	n = 200 100% women (50% breast cancer, 50% without cancer)	Chemotherapy treatment	Case-control observational	To analyze and compare foot health and general health in a sample of women with breast cancer and healthy women.	Foot Health Status Questionnaire and podiatric assessment	Yes	Yes	• *Foot health problems* Women with breast cancer reported 94% of foot problems. The most frequent alterations in the feet were: nail abnormalities (46%), pain (36%), cracks and dryness (20%), paresthesia (19%), inflammation (10%), varices (8%), deformed fingers (7%), and helomas and hardness (4%). Other problems reported were cramps, loss of sensation, or blisters. • *Foot health problems related to QoL* Women with breast cancer have a lower foot health-related QoL compared with healthy women. Clinical aspects, with an emphasis on foot pain and disability, were increased. Physical activity, social capacity, and vigor were affected. Therefore, more attention should be paid to the general health care and prevention of foot problems in breast cancer survivors.

Table 2. Cont.

First Author, Year, Country (Health Professional Department)	Journal	Sample	Anticancer Therapies	Type of Study	Research Objectives	Data Collection Methods Concerning Foot	Was the Aim of the Study the Foot Health?	Studied Foot Health Problems Related QoL	Main Findings
Engvall et al. [31], 2022, Sweden (Department of Oncology and Pharmacology)	Breast Cancer Research and Treatment	646 survivors of breast cancer	Post-taxane treatment	Cross-sectional cohort study	To explore the impact of persistent sensory and motor taxane-induced peripheral neuropathy symptoms on health-related QoL among early-stage breast cancer survivors.	EORTC QLQ-C30, HADS, CIPN20	Focused on peripheral neuropathy	Yes	• *Foot health problems related to QoL* TIPN has a significant impact on global QoL. The main important things were "difficulty walking because of foot drop" and "problems standing/walking because of difficulty feeling ground under feet". The authors reveal that although it is not usually life-threatening, it can significantly affect QoL.
Winther et al. [29], 2007, Denmark (Department of Oncology)	Supportive Care Cancer	$n = 55$ breast cancer	Chemotherapy treatment (docetaxel)	Observational and prevalence study	To estimate the frequency and severity of nail changes due to treatment.	NCICTCAE	No (nails, both hands and feet)	Yes	• *Foot health problems* A total of 88.5% reported changes in the nails after three cycles, 37.2% took place in the foot, 42.9% developed functional problems, and 37% had problems finding proper footwear. The association between nail changes and fungal infection was not found. They observed that the prevalence and aesthetic implications are similar in hands and feet, although the trend was higher in the hands. They found a statistically significant relationship between having neuropathy and nail changes in the feet ($p < 0.001$). • *Foot health problems related to QoL* Nail changes have both cosmetic and functional impact, which may lead to a decrease in QoL. A total of 28.6% presented mild functional problems, 8.6% moderate problems, and 5.7% severe problems due to nail changes.

Table 2. Cont.

First Author, Year, Country (Health Professional Department)	Journal	Sample	Anticancer Therapies	Type of Study	Research Objectives	Data Collection Methods Concerning Foot	Was the Aim of the Study the Foot Health?	Studied Foot Health Problems Related QoL	Main Findings
Monfort et al. [28], 2017, United States (Department of Oncology, biostatistics, engineering)	Breast Cancer Research and Treatment	n = 33 breast cancer patients (32 female/1 male)	Taxane	Longitudinal study	To describe symptoms of CIPN and functional impairments.	Standing balance, gait, Modified Total Neuropathy Score, Patient Report Outcomes (EORTC QLQ-CIPN20, EORTC QLQ-C30, BPI-SF)	No (peripheral neuropathy—gait)	Yes	• *Foot health problems* Significant negative changes were observed concerning gait, balance, and symptoms reported by people. A worsening of sensory, motor, and autonomic symptoms and pain has been reported with cumulative taxane exposure. They observed that, in the first cycle of chemotherapy, the balance was reduced in 28% of cases and walking speed in 5%. • *Foot health problems related to QoL.* Worsened physical functioning was shown on the EORTC QLQ-C30.
Biswal et al. [27], 2018, India (Department of Dermatology)	Indian Journal of Dermatology	n = 1000 Different tumor (24.1% genitourinary, 14.7% breast)	Chemotherapy drugs in combination (mostly alkylating agents)	Observational study	To know the cutaneous adversities in patients undergoing chemotherapy and the drug(s) most commonly associated with them.	Clinical manifestations	No (cutaneous adversities)	No	• *Foot health problems* Different cutaneous adversities of chemotherapy were found, such as xerosis (4.4%), melanonychia (2.9%), or HFS (2.6%). • *Foot health problems related to QoL.* It is pointed out that it is important to improve knowledge about adverse effects of anticancer drugs, which will help reduce psychological trauma and improve QoL.
Urakawa, et al. [26], 2019, Japan (Department of Dermatology and Pharmacology)	Journal of Cancer	n = 67 Cancer patients	Skin-toxic chemotherapeutic agents	Cross-sectional study	To investigate which skin toxicities influenced QoL and to what extent.	NCICTCAE, Dermatology Life Quality Index, and Skindex	No (skin toxicities)	Yes	• *Foot health problems* This research studied general skin toxicities. A total of 21 subjects developed paronychia, and 25 developed hand-foot syndrome. • *Foot health problems related to QoL.* HFS was a stronger factor in decreasing QOL than xerosis, paronychia, pigmentation, or rash. Therefore, especially in HFS, prevention, early detection, and daily medical care are necessary to maintain QOL.

BPI-SF: Brief Pain Inventory-Short Form; CIPN: Chemotherapy-Induced Peripheral Neuropathy; EORTC QLQ-CIPN 20: European Organization for Research and Treatment of Cancer Quality of Life Questionnaire-Chemotherapy-Induced Peripheral Neuropathy; EORTC QLQ-C30: European Organization for Research and Treatment of Cancer Quality of Life Questionnaire; DLA: Daily Living Activities; HADS: Hospital Anxiety and Depression Scale; HF QoLS: Hand-Foot Quality of Life Scale; HFS: Hand-Foot syndrome; NCICTCAE: National Cancer Institute Common Terminology Criteria for Adverse Events; QoL: quality of life; TIPN: Taxane-Induced Peripheral Neuropathy.

3.1. Bibliometric Characteristics

Most of the included studies were published in 2019 (n = 3) [24–26], 2018 (n = 2) [13,27], and 2017 (n = 2) [12,28]. The oldest articles are from 2007 [29] y 2009 [30]. Four papers were published in Asia [24–27], three in Europe [12,29,31], three in North America [13,28,32], and one in Australia [30].

The interdisciplinary contributions to the subject come mainly from the departments of oncology (n = 4) [13,28,29,31], nursing (n = 3) [12,24,25], pharmacy (n = 3) [26,30,31], and dermatology (n = 3) [26,27,32]. Only two articles involved professionals specializing in foot health or podiatry [12,13].

The most studied type of cancer was breast cancer. Most of the articles studied taxane-based chemotherapy. Mainly, the documents included are quantitative observational studies (n = 5) and reviews (n = 3). Only one work is a qualitative study.

3.2. Methods of Collecting Information about the Foot

Six papers used the National Cancer Institute's Common Terminology Criteria for Adverse Events. Two articles used scales related to hand–foot syndrome and QoL. The European Organization Peripheral Neuropathy Related QoL Scale was used in two investigations. Only one article used a specific questionnaire related to foot health and QoL (the Foot Health Status Questionnaire (FHSQ)), and another paper used in-depth interviews.

3.3. Main Objectives of the Documents Concerning the Foot

No study provided data on structural problems. Only one article addressed biomechanical problems (gait and balance) (Figure 2).

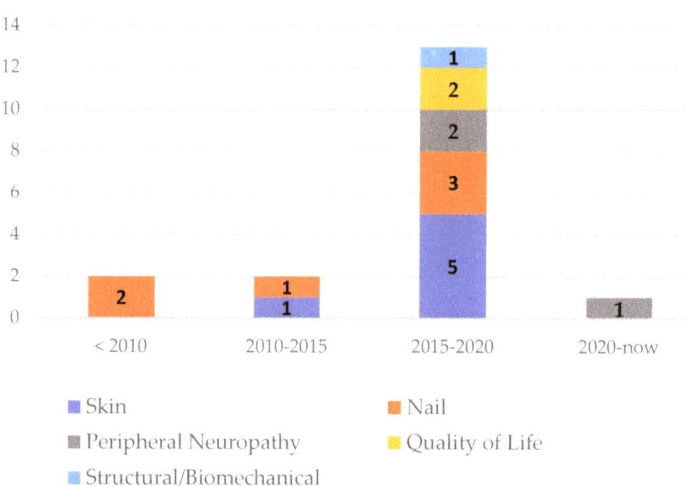

Figure 2. Main objectives of the documents concerning the foot/year of publication.

3.4. Findings from Thematic Analysis

The emerging themes of the analysis developed are shown below and in Table 2, which are not independent but are related to each other.

3.4.1. Foot Health Adverse Events

A significant number of the studies focused on nail and skin toxicities [12,13,26,27,29,30,32]. Biswal and Mehta [27] showed the association between toxicities and the type of chemotherapy and reported that: 2.6% presented hand–foot syndrome associated with docetaxel and antibodies; 2.9% melanonychia, associated with cisplatin and paclitaxel; and 4.4% xerosis, usually manifested with 5-Fluorouracil. Miller et al. [32]

reported that onycholysis arises from insults to the nail bed, is associated with taxanes, and has a prevalence of 0% to 44%. Beau's lines, subungual hemorrhage, nail pigmentation, paronychia, and splinter hemorrhages are also associated with this drug (up to 88% of subjects). The remainder of the publications focused solely on hand–foot syndrome [25,32], which was associated in 89% of cases with doxorubicin and 5-Fluorouracil [32].

Montfort et al. [28] published the only study that addressed gait in peripheral neuropathy. They observed a decrease in balance ($p = 0.001$) and speed ($p = 0.003$). Lacouture et al. [13] and López-Palomo et al. [12] were the only ones to directly describe foot health problems (Table 2).

3.4.2. Foot Health: A Critical Role Related to QoL of People Undergoing Anticancer Therapies

By focusing on foot health problems and using the analytic approaches mentioned above, the authors found that foot health problems related to QoL were highly highlighted in the included scientific literature. Consequently, this was a variable that emerged from the analysis of this study.

Thus, Palomo-López [12] studied podiatric adverse effects related to QoL among healthy women and those with breast cancer. Using the FHSQ, they observed significant differences in the domains of foot pain ($p = 0.003$), foot function ($p < 0.001$), physical activity ($p < 0.001$), social ability ($p < 0.001$), and vigor ($p < 0.001$)). Lacouture et al. [13] indicate that foot pain was scored at ≥ 8, and after the podiatry intervention, it improved to 4.8 ± 3.0 ($p < 0.001$). Similar results were obtained for QoL. Another study found that poorer QoL was also associated with decreased balance and walking speed ($p < 0.05$) [28].

Nail problems are associated with cosmetic problems, discomfort, pain, and impairment of QoL and activities of daily living [29–31], and can add morbidity and functional impairment [31]. On the other hand, Urakawa et al. [26] showed that the hand–foot syndrome had the highest statistically significant association with worse QoL ($p < 0.05$) among all the cutaneous adverse effects. Hsu et al. [25] observed that worse scores were obtained as the severity of toxicity increased ($p < 0.05$). In a qualitative study [24], participants identified this effect as a feeling of helplessness due to persistent symptoms. In addition, a body image problem arises since the appearance of the skin presents a dark coloration with a dirty appearance that they want to hide.

4. Discussion

The scientific evidence focused on foot health has grown significantly in the last 20 years, and the need for systematic reviews to develop evidence-based foot health science has been previously established [33]. The implications of foot health on QoL have been studied in other groups recently [34]. However, although cancer is a topic of great importance today and there is a lot of literature that addresses this health problem and the adverse effects of its therapies, there is a gap in the literature on its implications for foot health. The works found studied adverse effects in a general way or focused specifically and independently on any of them without focusing on foot health as a fundamental and determinant part of health [14].

This scoping review was conducted to illuminate to what extent foot health problems in people with cancer undergoing chemotherapy have been described in the literature. To the best of our knowledge, this is the first comprehensive review that attempts to address this issue. Only two articles addressed foot health, which were precisely the studies involving foot health professionals [12,13]. The information they provide suggests that their holistic study is essential since different organs are involved and have emotional, social, and physical consequences [34].

The lack of sufficient evidence did not allow us to compare information between studies nor to conclude to what extent and how it can be summarized in terms of foot problems related to QoL, this being the epicenter of future research. The description of foot health problems related to QoL in people with cancer undergoing chemotherapy is a theme and a variable that emerged from the first analysis of this scoping review. Foot health problems related to QoL were very prominent in all the papers articulated in the results, which allows us to have a more complete picture of this study area. Thus, QoL gained relevance, which is why it was included in the Results and Discussion sections. Overall, there has been a perceived gap in the literature since the development of the search strategy for this review. It is striking that the addition of the word "podiatry" did not yield results, which justifies the need to develop this area. Furthermore, it was surprising that the first articles were published in 2002, even though chemotherapy has been used for 80 years. Likewise, no research has been published in South America or Africa, despite the fact that the cancer data in these countries are overwhelming (11% increase in Africa and 101% increase in South America) [3].

It should be added that most of the public information that can be easily accessed is found in institutions such as the *National Cancer Institute*, the *American Cancer Society*, the *Spanish Society of Medical Oncology*, the *Canadian Cancer Society*, the *American Society of Clinical Oncology, Memorial Sloan Kettering Cancer Center*, the *Centers for Disease Control and Prevention, and Cancer Research UK*. These sources describe the adverse effects of cancer therapies. Only the National Cancer Institute includes information on skin and nail changes, although, like the reviewed literature, they only refer to the foot when describing hand–foot syndrome.

4.1. Literature Gap from the Foot Health Perspective: A Challenge for Discussion

Overall, the results showed that foot problems are relevant and impair wellbeing. Focused instruments on foot health were not thoroughly used. Mainly, scientific evidence addresses nail and skin problems. Initially, many articles were found, since the hand–foot syndrome is mentioned in many studies that address the adverse effects of treatments or their effectiveness [35]. However, they did not respond to the proposed objective. The oldest publications dealt with nail conditions. Since 2015, the evidence has covered a greater variety of topics (Figure 2). There was great disagreement about the magnitude of nail problems: while Gilbar et al. [30] mention that it is a practically unknown problem, Winther et al. [29] indicate that 88.5% present nail problems after three cycles of chemotherapy. Likewise, Zawar et al. [36] report that the most frequent nail changes were color change (54.26%) and nail dystrophy (29.45%), citing them as common effects. Instead, Miller et al. [32] reported other problems, such as onycholysis, with data ranging from 0% to 44%. They all agree that these conditions have received little attention in the oncology community. Furthermore, they indicate that much of the literature consists of case studies published in dermatology journals [30].

Regarding skin problems, 90% of people experience them at some point during treatment [37]. Hand-foot syndrome was very prominent in the results of this review [24,25], which is consistent with published evidence [38]. It is indicated that this condition had the highest degree of toxicity after the hematological one (25% of the cases). Alizadeh et al. [38] indicate that it occurs mainly between the third and sixth cycles of chemotherapy, which is consistent with the results presented. In addition, it is defined as a relevant cause for the suspension or limitation of treatment [39–41].

On the other hand, there is wide-ranging literature on the pathophysiological mechanisms of peripheral neuropathy. Although the foot is the most affected part, there is no literature that specifically focuses on what happens in the lower extremity [42]. By contrast, there is research on its involvement in QoL, gait, and balance [28]. Furthermore, a study [31] focused on QoL used scales that involved items related to the foot, which were the most prominent and negatively associated with QoL. It is noteworthy that no research has alluded to diabetes when the evidence points to it as a risk factor for peripheral neuropathy [43].

Lastly, Palomo-López [12] compared a sample of healthy women with breast cancer and chemotherapy, and Lacouture et al. [13] reported the clinical experience of the Oncology Department of a hospital in the Netherlands. They constitute the only works that revealed the implications of chemotherapy in the foot globally. They report problems such as hyperkeratosis (4%), xerosis (20%), digital deformities (7%), and paresthesias (19%), data that attract attention due to their low proportion. These studies focused on foot health report a greater diversity of effects, unlike the rest of the works included, which mostly only mentioned hand–foot syndrome or neuropathy. This agrees with two reports published in the United Kingdom. They describe some podiatric adverse effects that have been poorly described from a foot health perspective [44,45].

4.2. QoL of People with Cancer: An Agenda That Should Consider Foot Health

Cancer constitutes a threat to the wellbeing and perception of an individual's QoL [46]. The increase in cancer survivors and the toxic effects of treatment that emerge during and after treatment have placed QoL in the critical focus of attention [47]. Although most toxicities are not the cause of a person's death, they are critical to receiving treatment, enjoying adequate QoL during and after the disease process, and avoiding the loss of years of healthy life [31].

Even though no research has been found that addresses the implications that podiatric adverse effects have on QoL in a specific way, most of the included studies alluded to the negative contribution of these problems to people's wellbeing and health. Only one article used a questionnaire that focused on foot health related to the person's QoL [12] and not on each individual symptom. Therefore, we cannot compare this information with other studies, and we cannot conclude to what extent and how people's QoL is influenced by podiatric adverse effects.

Winther et al. [29] found that 28.6% had mild, 8.6% moderate, and 5.7% severe functional problems due to nail changes. It affects one cosmetically and functionally and leads to a decrease in QoL. Although the data were not consistent between the included studies, they agreed that these problems were debilitating [38]. Regarding hand–foot syndrome, the included papers [24–26] mainly addressed its implications for QoL and daily activities. In the literature, a specific questionnaire was even found that assessed this aspect [48]. This effect stands out especially because it can severely present itself and lead to the suspension of chemotherapy, as shown by some case studies [49]. For this reason, new theories are emerging regarding this adverse effect, including the need for prevention, early detection, and daily care to maintain QoL and avoid further implications in the disease process, such as dose modification [26]. In addition, it is a prominent factor because it contributes to physical inactivity and falls [49].

Ganz and Dougherty [47] reflect on the importance of toxicities that emerge during treatment and after its completion, highlighting peripheral neuropathy due to its difficulty in managing even today. This agrees with other investigations [7], which report a correlation between adverse effects such as neuropathy and edema and a decrease in QoL. Other recent research shows that foot assessment methods are inconsistent among published studies, that the effects of neuropathy on foot health are most prominent, and that it adds morbidity to the cancer population [42]. Like hand–foot syndrome, this effect is associated with falls and balance problems [49]. Other literature states that neuropathy is associated with anxiety, depression, insomnia, and falls ($p < 0.05$) [50,51]. Finally, a point to note is that after treatment, problems such as neuropathy can be persistent and favor barriers related to sensorimotor and mobility deficits. This is associated with the possibility of not performing physical activity, decreased ambulation, and an increased body mass index, which may be correlated with other health problems [28,51].

4.3. Future Lines of Research and Clinical Practice

Future research should deepen knowledge about the influence of podiatric adverse effects on QoL in people with cancer undergoing chemotherapy. It is necessary to articulate research in other tumors, both sexes and other geographical locations. The current dearth of scientific evidence is linked to the fact that these effects are neglected in current oncological clinical practice. Only institutions and societies make indirect reference to these effects, but without focusing on the foot. This invites us to focus on this agenda from a comprehensive and holistic perspective, advancing research while providing guidelines through clinical practice guidelines. In addition, the fact that only the articles focused on foot health were carried out by healthcare professionals such as podiatrists and that the inclusion of the word "podiatry" in the search strategy did not produce any results justifies the need for these professionals to form part of the oncology work team.

What has been described above is related to the need to contribute to the current focus of attention for people with cancer: QoL. For that purpose, it is necessary to respond to a part of the knowledge that has not been described up to now. The need to: (a) develop standardized methods and specialized professionals for the assessment of the foot is evident, since their absence can hide the presence of podiatric problems; and (b) get involved in the symptom and attend to it through standardized guidelines [52]. In this sense, in addition to education on how to care for the foot and control symptoms, it is necessary to educate people about the adverse effects of anticancer drugs that people can develop, which will help with psychological trauma and improve QoL [27].

Particularly, hand–foot syndrome is the only dermal toxicity that does not present prevention or current treatment guidelines, despite being the most prevalent side effect, and that is related to a greater impact on QoL and dose limitation. Knowing that managing these effects can minimize treatment interruptions and improve people's wellbeing, future research should focus on this aspect [53,54].

Clinical practice should be directed towards the prevention, diagnosis, and management of podiatric adverse events as an essential part of foot function and health-related quality of life and as an integral part of care, critical aspects for the care of people with cancer and survivors [13,26,40].

Consistent with what was observed in this study, in 2017, Lacouture et al. [13] reported that no podiatric screening and treatment have been developed to prevent or mitigate podiatric adverse events in cancer patients. As they described, a foot care program must include topics such as QoL and risk factors. Concerning peripheral neuropathy, recent research reports on the main complementary therapies to prevent or treat this side effect. It stands out in the exercise [42]. Concerning nail and dermal toxicities, such as paronychia or hand–foot syndrome, topical antibiotics, or urea cream [13].

Overall, the achievement of these improvements in practice must be based on person-centered care and a biopsychosocial approach. It is necessary that professionals, such as nurses and podiatrists, work together based on multidimensional interventions and person-centered self-care [55]. Nurses are in close contact with people, so the guidance provided during care will be essential. For this, it is necessary to listen to the demands and complaints of people in order to develop sensitive prevention and treatment strategies that are appropriate to their needs [47].

Therefore, the application of what is described in this review will guide not only professionals specialized in foot health but also oncologists, nurses, and especially the people themselves and their relatives/caregivers.

5. Conclusions

This research is the first to focus on foot health as a fundamental part of the quality of life of people with cancer undergoing chemotherapy. So far, no study has focused specifically on a sample of people with cancer receiving chemotherapy, and there is not sufficient information on how QoL is influenced by these adverse effects, which should be the epicenter of future investigations.

This study provides new insight into foot health, whose problems are diverse and relevant. Specifically, the problems described seem to favor people's disabilities and affect activities of daily living. In addition, they imply the possibility of limiting or suspending the treatment dose, which highlights the problem analyzed. More studies are needed to contribute to the care of people with cancer through foot health.

Author Contributions: Conceptualization, design, planning, methodology, validation, R.V.-S. and C.G.-M.; writing—original draft preparation, R.V.-S.; supervision, C.G.-M. All authors have read and agreed to the published version of the manuscript.

Funding: The APC was funded by the Instituto de Investigación Biomédica de A Coruña (INIBIC).

Institutional Review Board Statement: Not applicable.

Informed Consent Statement: Not applicable.

Data Availability Statement: Not applicable.

Acknowledgments: This work was supported by a fellow scholarship of Raquel Veiga-Seijo, by financing from the Sistema Gallego de Universidades with the European Social Fund 2014–2020, and by the Secretaría Xeral Universidades of Galicia with the reference ED481A-2020/034. We would like to thank the staff of the Oza Library of the University of A Coruña for their help.

Conflicts of Interest: The authors declare no conflict of interest.

References

1. National Cancer Institute. What Is Cancer? 2015. Available online: https://www.cancer.gov/about-cancer/understanding/what-is-cancer (accessed on 1 December 2022).
2. World Health Organization. Cancer. 2018. Available online: https://www.who.int/es/news-room/fact-sheets/detail/cancer (accessed on 1 December 2022).
3. Siegel, R.L.; Miller, K.D.; Wagle, N.S.; Jemal, A. Cancer statistics. *CA Cancer J. Clin.* **2023**, *73*, 17–48. [CrossRef] [PubMed]
4. Sung, H.; Ferlay, J.; Siegel, R.L.; Laversanne, M.; Soerjomataram, I.; Jemal, A.; Bray, F. Global cancer statistics 2020: Globocan estimates of incidence and mortality worldwide for 36 cancers in 185 countries. *CA Cancer J. Clin.* **2021**, *71*, 209–249. [CrossRef] [PubMed]
5. Emine, K.E.; Gulbeyaz, C. The effect of salt-water bath in the management of treatment-related peripheral neuropathy in cancer patients receiving taxane and platinum-based treatment. *Explore* **2022**, *18*, 347–356. [CrossRef]
6. Kocarnik, J.M.; Compton, K.; Dean, F.E.; Fu, W.; Gaw, B.L.; Harvey, J.D.; Henrikson, H.J.; Lu, D.; Pennini, A.; Xu, R.; et al. Cancer Incidence, Mortality, Years of Life Lost, Years Lived with Disability, and Disability-Adjusted Life Years for 29 Cancer Groups From 2010 to 2019 A Systematic Analysis for the Global Burden of Disease Study 2019. *JAMA Oncol.* **2022**, *8*, 420–444. [PubMed]
7. Hirose, C.; Fujii, H.; Iihara, H.; Ishihara, M.; Nawa-Nishigaki, M.; Kato-Hayashi, H.; Ohata, K.; Sekiya, K.; Kitahora, M.; Matsuhashi, N.; et al. Real-world data of the association between quality of life using the EuroQol 5 Dimension 5 Level utility value and adverse events for outpatient cancer chemotherapy. *Support. Care Cancer* **2020**, *28*, 5943–5952. [CrossRef]
8. Tachi, T.; Teramachi, H.; Tanaka, K.; Asano, S.; Osawa, T.; Kawashima, A.; Yasuda, M.; Mizui, T.; Nakada, T.; Noguchi, Y.; et al. The impact of outpatient chemotherapy-related adverse events on the quality of life of breast cancer patients. *PLoS ONE* **2015**, *10*, e0124169. [CrossRef]
9. Hagiwara, Y.; Shiroiwa, T.; Shimozuma, K.; Kawahara, T.; Uemura, Y.; Watanabe, T.; Taira, N.; Fukuda, T.; Ohashi, Y.; Mukai, H. Impact of Adverse Events on Health Utility and Health-Related Quality of Life in Patients Receiving First-Line Chemotherapy for Metastatic Breast Cancer: Results from the SELECT BC Study. *Pharmacoeconomics* **2018**, *36*, 215–223. [CrossRef]
10. Stolt, M. Individual's Foot Health. In *Individualized Care: Theory, Measurement, Research and Practice*, 1st ed.; Springer: Berlin/Heidelberg, Germany, 2019; pp. 163–169.
11. Stolt, M.; Gattinger, H.; Boström, C.; Suhonen, R. Foot health educational interventions for patients and healthcare professionals: A scoping review. *Health Educ. J.* **2019**, *79*, 390–416. [CrossRef]
12. López, P.P.; Rodríguez-Sanz, D.; Vallejo, R.B.D.B.; Losa-Iglesias, M.E.; Martín, J.G.; Lobo, C.C.; Lopez, D.L. Clinical aspects of foot health and their influence on quality of life among breast cancer survivors: A case–control study. *Cancer Manag. Res.* **2017**, *9*, 545–551. [CrossRef]
13. Lacouture, M.E.; Kopsky, D.J.; Lilker, R.; Damstra, F.; van der Linden, M.H.M.; Freites-Martinez, A.; Nagel, M.P.M. Podiatric Adverse Events and Foot Care in Cancer Patients and Survivors Awareness, Education, and Literature Review. *J. Am. Podiatr. Med. Assoc.* **2018**, *108*, 508–516. [CrossRef]
14. Brodie, B.S. Health determinants and podiatry. *Perspect. Public Health* **2001**, *121*, 174–176. [CrossRef] [PubMed]
15. Edwards, K.; Borthwick, A.; McCulloch, L.; Redmond, A.; Pinedo-Villanueva, R.; Prieto-Alhambra, D.; Judge, A.; Arden, N.; Bowen, C. Evidence for current recommendations concerning the management of foot health for people with chronic long-term conditions: A systematic review. *J. Foot Ankle Res.* **2017**, *10*, 51. [CrossRef] [PubMed]
16. Williams, A.E.; Graham, A.S. 'My feet-visible, but ignored.' A qualitative study of foot care for people with rheumatoid arthritis. *Clin. Rehabil.* **2012**, *26*, 952–959. [CrossRef] [PubMed]
17. Lazzarini, P.A.; Hurn, S.; Kuys, S.; Kamp, M.C.; Ng, V.; Thomas, C.; Jen, S.; Kinnear, E.M.; D'Emden, M.C.; Reed, L. Direct inpatient burden caused by foot-related conditions: A multisite point-prevalence study. *BMJ Open* **2016**, *6*, e010811. [CrossRef]
18. Laitinen, A.-M.; Boström, C.; Hyytiä, S.; Stolt, M. Experiences of foot health in patients with rheumatoid arthritis: A qualitative study. *Disabil. Rehabil.* **2020**, *44*, 88–95. [CrossRef]

19. Arksey, H.; O'Malley, L. Scoping studies: Towards a methodological framework. *Int. J. Soc. Res. Methodol.* **2005**, *8*, 19–32. [CrossRef]
20. Tricco, A.C.; Lillie, E.; Zarin, W.; O'Brien, K.K.; Colquhoun, H.; Levac, D.; Moher, D.; Peters, M.D.J.; Horsley, T.; Weeks, L.; et al. PRISMA extension for scoping reviews (PRISMA-ScR): Checklist and explanation. *Ann. Intern. Med.* **2018**, *169*, 467–473. [CrossRef]
21. Levac, D.; Colquhoun, H.; O'Brien, K.K. Scoping studies: Advancing the methodology. *Implement. Sci.* **2010**, *5*, 69. [CrossRef]
22. Peters, M.; Godfrey, C.; McInerney, P.; Munn, Z.; Trico, A.; Khalil, H. Chapter 11: Scoping Reviews. In *JBI Manual for Evidence Synthesis*; Aromataris, E., Munn, Z., Eds.; JBI: Long Beach, CA, USA, 2020.
23. Braun, V.; Clarke, V. Using thematic analysis in psychology. *Qual. Res. Psychol.* **2006**, *3*, 77–101. [CrossRef]
24. Komatsu, H.; Yagasaki, K.; Hirata, K.; Hamamoto, Y. Unmet needs of cancer patients with chemotherapy-related hand-foot syndrome and targeted therapy-related hand-foot skin reaction: A qualitative study. *Eur. J. Oncol. Nurs.* **2018**, *38*, 65–69. [CrossRef]
25. Hsu, Y.-H.; Shen, W.-C.; Wang, C.-H.; Lin, Y.-F.; Chen, S.-C. Hand-foot syndrome and its impact on daily activities in breast cancer patients receiving docetaxel-based chemotherapy. *Eur. J. Oncol. Nurs.* **2019**, *43*, 101670. [CrossRef] [PubMed]
26. Urakawa, R.; Tarutani, M.; Kubota, K.; Uejima, E. Hand Foot Syndrome Has the Strongest Impact on QOL in Skin Toxicities of Chemotherapy. *J. Cancer* **2019**, *10*, 4846–4851. [CrossRef] [PubMed]
27. Biswal, S.G.; Mehta, R.D. Cutaneous Adverse Reactions of Chemotherapy in Cancer Patients: A Clinicoepidemiological Study. *Indian J. Dermatol.* **2018**, *63*, 41–46. [CrossRef] [PubMed]
28. Monfort, S.M.; Pan, X.; Patrick, R.; Ramaswamy, B.; Wesolowski, R.; Naughton, M.J.; Loprinzi, C.L.; Chaudhari, A.M.W.; Lustberg, M.B. Gait, balance, and patient-reported outcomes during taxane-based chemotherapy in early-stage breast cancer patients. *Breast Cancer Res. Treat.* **2017**, *164*, 69–77. [CrossRef]
29. Winther, D.; Saunte, D.M.; Knap, M.; Haahr, V.; Jensen, A.B. Nail changes due to docetaxel—A neglected side effect and nuisance for the patient. *Support. Care Cancer* **2007**, *15*, 1191–1197. [CrossRef] [PubMed]
30. Gilbar, P.; Hain, A.; Peereboom, V.-M. Nail Toxicity Induced by Cancer Chemotherapy. *J. Oncol. Pharm. Pract.* **2009**, *15*, 143–155. [CrossRef]
31. Engvall, K.; Gréen, H.; Fredrikson, M.; Lagerlund, M.; Lewin, F.; Åvall-Lundqvist, E. Impact of persistent peripheral neuropathy on health-related quality of life among early-stage breast cancer survivors: A population-based cross-sectional study. *Breast Cancer Res. Treat.* **2022**, *195*, 379–391. [CrossRef]
32. Miller, K.K.; Gorcey, L.; McLellan, B.N. Chemotherapy-induced hand-foot syndrome and nail changes: A review of clinical presentation, etiology, pathogenesis, and management. *J. Am. Acad. Dermatol.* **2014**, *71*, 787–794. [CrossRef]
33. Hawke, F.; Burns, J.; Landorf, K.B. Evidence-based podiatric medicine. *J. Am. Podiatr. Med. Assoc.* **2009**, *99*, 260–266. [CrossRef]
34. López-López, D.; Pérez-Ríos, M.; Ruano-Ravina, A.; Losa-Iglesias, M.E.; Becerro-De-Bengoa-Vallejo, R.; Romero-Morales, C.; Calvo-Lobo, C.; Navarro-Flores, E. Impact of quality of life related to foot problems: A case–control study. *Sci. Rep.* **2021**, *11*, 1–6. [CrossRef]
35. Grenon, N.N. Managing toxicities associated with antiangiogenic biologic agents in combination with chemotherapy for metastatic colorectal cancer. *Clin. J. Oncol. Nurs.* **2013**, *17*, 425–433. [CrossRef] [PubMed]
36. Zawar, V.; Bondarde, S.; Pawar, M.; Sankalecha, S. Nail changes due to chemotherapy: A prospective observational study of 129 patients. *J. Eur. Acad. Dermatol. Venereol.* **2019**, *33*, 1398–1404. [CrossRef] [PubMed]
37. Ding, J.F.; Farah, M.H.; Nayfeh, T.; Malandris, K.; Manolopoulos, A.; Ginex, P.K.; Hasan, B.; Dunnack, H.; Abd-Rabu, R.; Rajjoub, M.R.; et al. Targeted Therapy– and Chemotherapy-Associated Skin Toxicities: Systematic Review and Meta-Analysis. *Oncol. Nurs. Forum* **2020**, *47*, E149–E160. [CrossRef] [PubMed]
38. Alizadeh, N.; Mirpour, S.H.; Darjani, A.; Rafiei, R.; Rafiei, E.; Mohammadhoseini, M. Dermatologic adverse effects of breast cancer chemotherapy: A longitudinal prospective observational study with a review of literature. *Int. J. Dermatol.* **2020**, *59*, 822–828. [CrossRef]
39. Lambert-Falls, R.; Modugno, S. Toxicity of dose-dense docetaxel followed by doxorubicin with cyclophosphamide as adjuvant therapy for breast cancer in a phase II study. *Clin. Breast Cancer* **2007**, *7*, 697–704. [CrossRef]
40. Viale, P.H. Chemotherapy and Cutaneous Toxicities: Implications for Oncology Nurses. *Semin. Oncol. Nurs.* **2006**, *22*, 144–151. [CrossRef]
41. Zaiem, A.; Hammamia, S.; Aouinti, I.; Charfi, O.; Ladhari, W.; Kastalli, S.; El Aidli, S.; Lakhoua, G. Hand-foot syndrome induced by chemotherapy drug: Case series study and literature review. *Indian J. Pharmacol.* **2022**, *54*, 208–215.
42. Veiga-Seijo, R.; Perez-Lopez, M.E.; Fernandez-Lopez, U.; Mosquera-Fernandez, A.; Seijo-Bestilleiro, R.; Gonzalez-Martin, C. Wellbeing and Complementary Therapies in Breast Cancer Peripheral Neuropathy Care: A Scoping Review Focused on Foot Health. *Cancers* **2023**, *15*, 2110. [CrossRef]
43. Gu, J.; Lu, H.; Chen, C.; Gu, Z.; Hu, M.; Liu, L.; Yu, J.; Wei, G.; Huo, J. Diabetes mellitus as a risk factor for chemotherapy-induced peripheral neuropathy: A meta-analysis. *Support. Care Cancer* **2021**, *29*, 7461–7469. [CrossRef]
44. Shah-Hamilton, A. The impact of anti-cancer treatment on feet. Podiatric Adverse Events: Part 2a Neurological Effects. *Podiatry Rev.* **2021**, *2*, 26–29.
45. Shah-Hamilton, A. The impact of anti-cancer treatment on feet. Podiatric Adverse Events: Part 2b Dermatological Effects. *Podiatry Rev.* **2021**, *1*, 32–36.

46. Rustøen, T. Hope and quality of life, two central issues for cancer patients: A theoretical analysis. *Cancer Nurs.* **1995**, *18*, 355–361. Available online: http://www.ncbi.nlm.nih.gov/pubmed/7585489 (accessed on 1 December 2022). [PubMed]
47. Ganz, P.A.; Dougherty, P.M. Painful Hands and Feet After Cancer Treatment: Inflammation Affecting the Mind-Body Connection. *J. Clin. Oncol.* **2016**, *34*, 649–652. [CrossRef] [PubMed]
48. Anderson, R.T.; Keating, K.N.; Doll, H.A.; Camacho, F. The Hand-Foot Skin Reaction and Quality of Life Questionnaire: An Assessment Tool for Oncology. *Oncologist* **2015**, *20*, 831–838. [CrossRef] [PubMed]
49. Dar, W.; Hussain, M.; Aziz, S.A.; Mohammad, G.; Wani, B.; Latief, M. Uncommon adverse effects of commonly used chemotherapeutic agents in medical oncology practice: A series of two cases of hand-foot syndrome. *Indian. J. Med. Paediatr. Oncol.* **2017**, *38*, 380–382. [CrossRef]
50. Bao, T.; Basal, C.; Seluzicki, C.; Li, S.Q.; Seidman, A.D.; Mao, J.J. Long-term chemotherapy-induced peripheral neuropathy among breast cancer survivors: Prevalence, risk factors, and fall risk. *Breast Cancer Res. Treat.* **2016**, *159*, 327–333. [CrossRef]
51. Mizrahi, D.; Goldstein, D.; Trinh, T.; Li, T.; Timmins, H.C.; Harrison, M.; Marx, G.M.; Hovey, E.J.; Lewis, C.R.; Friedlander, M.; et al. Physical activity behaviors in cancer survivors treated with neurotoxic chemotherapy. *Asia-Pac. J. Clin. Oncol.* **2022**, *19*, 243–249. [CrossRef]
52. Simsek, N.Y.; Demir, A. Cold Application and Exercise on Development of Peripheral Neuropathy during Taxane Chemotherapy in Breast Cancer Patients: A Randomized Controlled Trial. *Asia-Pac. J. Oncol. Nurs.* **2021**, *8*, 255–268. [CrossRef]
53. Williams, L.A.; Ginex, P.K.; Ebanks, G.L.; Ganstwig, K.; Ciccolini, K.; Kwong, B.Y.; Robison, J.; Shelton, G.; Strelo, J.; Wiley, K.; et al. ONS guidelines™ for cancer treatment-related skin toxicity. *Oncol. Nurs. Forum.* **2020**, *47*, 539–556. [CrossRef]
54. Velasco, R.; Navarro, X.; Gil-Gil, M.; Herrando-Grabulosa, M.; Calls, A.; Bruna, J. Neuropathic Pain and Nerve Growth Factor in Chemotherapy-Induced Peripheral Neuropathy: Prospective Clinical-Pathological Study. *J. Pain. Symptom Manag.* **2017**, *54*, 815–825. [CrossRef]
55. Kevin, D.; Brabants, A.; Nester, C.; Gijon-Nogueron, G.; Simşek, E.; Newton, V. A conceptual framework for contemporary professional foot care practice: "The value based digital foot care framework". *J. Foot Ankle Res.* **2021**, *14*, 22. [CrossRef]

Disclaimer/Publisher's Note: The statements, opinions and data contained in all publications are solely those of the individual author(s) and contributor(s) and not of MDPI and/or the editor(s). MDPI and/or the editor(s) disclaim responsibility for any injury to people or property resulting from any ideas, methods, instructions or products referred to in the content.

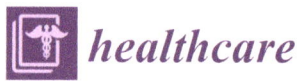

Article

Cancer Patients' Satisfaction with In-Home Palliative Care and Its Impact on Disease Symptoms

Inmaculada Valero-Cantero [1], Cristina Casals [2,*], Milagrosa Espinar-Toledo [3], Francisco Javier Barón-López [4], Francisco Javier Martínez-Valero [5] and María Ángeles Vázquez-Sánchez [6]

[1] Puerta Blanca Clinical Management Unit, Malaga-Guadalhorce Health District, 29004 Malaga, Spain
[2] ExPhy Research Group, Department of Physical Education, Instituto de Investigación e Innovación Biomédica de Cádiz (INiBICA), Universidad de Cádiz, 11519 Puerto Real, Spain
[3] Rincón de la Victoria Clinical Management Unit, Malaga-Guadalhorce Health District, 29730 Malaga, Spain
[4] Faculty of Health Sciences, Institute of Biomedical Research in Málaga (IBIMA), University of Malaga, 29016 Malaga, Spain
[5] Midlothian Foot Care, Dalkeith and National Health Service, Dalkeith EH22 1DU, UK
[6] Department of Nursing, Faculty of Health Sciences, PASOS Research Group and UMA REDIAS Network of Law and Artificial Intelligence Applied to Health and Biotechnology, University of Malaga, 29071 Malaga, Spain
* Correspondence: cristina.casals@uca.es

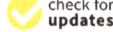

Abstract: The aim of the study was to determine whether the satisfaction of cancer patients with in-home palliative care is associated with the impact of disease symptoms and with self-perceived quality of life. This was a cross-sectional descriptive study, conducted in the primary health care sector in six clinical management units, where 72 patients were recruited over a period of six months. The severity of symptoms was determined by the Edmonton Symptom Assessment System (ESAS). Quality of life was evaluated with the EORTC QLQ-C30 (version 3) questionnaire, and patients' satisfaction with the care received was evaluated by the Client Satisfaction Questionnaire (CSQ-8). The patients' satisfaction with the health care received was represented by an average score of 6, on a scale of 1–10; thus, there is room for improvement in patient satisfaction. Moreover, it was found that more intense symptoms and lower quality of life are associated with lower satisfaction with health care received ($p = 0.001$). Similarly, when symptoms are more severe, the quality of life is lower ($p < 0.001$). The identification of fatigue, reduced well-being, pain, drowsiness, and depression as the symptoms experienced with the highest intensity by our patients provides valuable information for health care providers in developing individualized symptom management plans for patients with advanced cancer.

Keywords: medical oncology; quality of life; patient satisfaction; symptom assessment; palliative care; home care services; community health nursing

Citation: Valero-Cantero, I.; Casals, C.; Espinar-Toledo, M.; Barón-López, F.J.; Martínez-Valero, F.J.; Vázquez-Sánchez, M.Á. Cancer Patients' Satisfaction with In-Home Palliative Care and Its Impact on Disease Symptoms. *Healthcare* **2023**, *11*, 1272. https://doi.org/10.3390/healthcare11091272

Academic Editor: Qiuping Li

Received: 4 April 2023
Revised: 26 April 2023
Accepted: 27 April 2023
Published: 29 April 2023

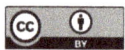

Copyright: © 2023 by the authors. Licensee MDPI, Basel, Switzerland. This article is an open access article distributed under the terms and conditions of the Creative Commons Attribution (CC BY) license (https://creativecommons.org/licenses/by/4.0/).

1. Introduction

Worldwide, cancer is a major cause of mortality, responsible for one in every six deaths, according to the World Health Organization [1]. Patients with advanced cancer need palliative care as early as possible [2,3], since they present changeable, severe symptoms that require continuous, high-quality health care [4]. This highlights the need for increased awareness and resources to be dedicated to palliative care for cancer patients.

Among other symptoms, patients may experience pain, fatigue, nausea, depression, anxiety, drowsiness, dyspnoea, sleep disorders, loss of appetite, constipation, and altered quality of life [5–8], and these symptoms usually worsen as the disease progresses [9]. Palliative care is aimed at relieving these symptoms and improving the patient's quality of life, as well as providing support for their families and caregivers, by addressing their physical, psychological, social, and spiritual needs.

In order to provide effective symptom management and improve the quality of life for patients with advanced cancer, healthcare providers must have reliable and accurate measures of the symptoms they are experiencing. The mentioned symptoms can be measured in various ways, but one of the most widely used instruments, both in clinical practice and in research, is the Edmonton Symptom Assessment Scale (ESAS) [10–12], which evaluates the intensity of ten physical and psychological symptoms. A major advantage of this scale is its ease of use [13]. Given the significant impact that advanced cancer and its related symptoms have on patients' well-being, it is essential that healthcare providers prioritize the regular assessment of symptoms in their care management plans.

One of the fundamental objectives of health care for these patients is to improve their quality of life, which is inevitably diminished by the oncological process and the symptoms produced [14]. Quality of life is a multidimensional construct that encompasses various aspects of an individual's life, including physical health, mental health, social functioning, and general well-being [15]. It is a subjective measure that reflects an individual's perception of their overall life satisfaction. Thus, assessing the patient's quality of life should be also an integral part of their overall health care management.

Quality health care should alleviate the symptoms (or at least maintain the status quo, or slow the worsening) presented by a cancer patient in palliative care, and hence improve the quality of life. However, to decide whether this care is really effective, the patient's own assessment of outcomes must be obtained, and this aspect of the question has received relatively little research attention [16]. Patient-reported outcomes have become increasingly important in assessing the effectiveness of health care interventions and should be considered in the evaluation of palliative care for cancer patients.

A further consideration is the fact that the patient's preferences in health care planning should be taken into account in the clinical setting. In this respect, some recommendations have already been offered [17]. The recommendations involve tailoring advance care planning to the readiness of the individual, adjusting the content of advance care planning as the individual's health condition worsens, and utilizing trained non-physician facilitators to support the advance care planning process [17]. Patients' satisfaction with the health care received is of fundamental importance and is closely related to the degree of concordance between the actual treatment and care received and the patient's preferences in this regard [18], and this consideration is as valid for patients receiving in-home palliative care as for those who are hospitalized [19].

On the other hand, according to prior research in the area of palliative care, advance health care planning between physicians and patients does not increase the latter's satisfaction with the medical care received [20], nor does it produce differences in treatment, in perceived quality of life, or in physical and mental symptoms [21]. In consequence, joint planning of the health care program between physicians and patients may not be strictly necessary. Nevertheless, an assessment of the patient's continuing acceptance of the treatment and care received may be useful, and this question can be assessed by means of user satisfaction surveys.

Our study aim is to determine whether satisfaction with the health care received is associated with the severity of symptoms and with self-perceived quality of life for patients with advanced cancer receiving in-home palliative care. The results of this study can be used to inform health care providers on how to improve care for advanced cancer patients receiving in-home palliative care, with the aim of improving patients' satisfaction, reducing the severity of symptoms, and enhancing their quality of life.

2. Materials and Methods

2.1. Design

The study employed a multicenter, cross-sectional descriptive design. It was conducted in the field of primary health care in six clinical management units in the Málaga-Guadalhorce Health District (Málaga, Andalusia, Spain).

2.2. Eligibility Criteria and Sampling

The following inclusion criteria were applied: (1) Cancer patients receiving in-home palliative care, (2) who were aged 18 years or older. The exclusion criteria were: (1) Patients with highly advanced disease, resulting in a life expectancy of only a few days, or (2) patients with advanced stage dementia or psychological disorders that would impair their ability to make rational decisions. All individuals included in the study had previously received treatment for cancer through surgery, radiotherapy, or chemotherapy. At the time of the study, none of the patients were receiving systemic treatment, and the treatment provided was focused on symptom improvement.

The study sample was constituted from the cancer patients who according to the corresponding Digital Clinical History (DIRAYA, Spanish initials) were currently receiving palliative care. DIRAYA, defined as an integrated management and information system for health care, is the system used in the Andalusian Health Service as a support for electronic medical records.

2.3. Measures

Several measures were utilized to collect data from participants, which were carefully selected based on their validity and reliability. The measures used in the present study are detailed as presented below.

2.3.1. Sociodemographic Data and Clinical Characteristics

The sociodemographic information included: age, sex, marital status, and education. The clinical characteristics included: type of cancer and duration of palliative care. This information was recorded to describe the study sample and consider the generalizability of the findings.

2.3.2. Severity of Disease Symptoms

Assessment of symptoms was conducted using the Edmonton Symptom Assessment System (ESAS) scale [10,22]. ESAS has been psychometrically validated and translated into over 20 languages with good internal reliability (Cronbach α 0.79), test-retest reliability (Spearman correlation coefficient 0.86 on Day 2 and 0.45 on Day 7), and convergent validity [10]. Moreover, the ESAS is a valid, reliable, responsive, and feasible instrument with adequate psychometric properties when tested on Spanish advanced cancer patients [23].

This instrument measures the average intensity of ten common symptoms experienced by cancer patients during the previous week. These symptoms include pain, fatigue, nausea, depression, anxiety, drowsiness, dyspnea, loss of appetite, reduced well-being, and sleep disorders. Patients rated the severity of each symptom at the time of evaluation on a scale from 0 to 10, where 0 indicates the symptom was absent and 10 that it was of the worst possible severity. Based on the ESAS symptoms, following outcomes were obtained:

- Physical ESAS score: calculated as the sum of pain, fatigue, nausea, drowsiness, appetite, and dyspnea symptoms (ranging from 0 to 60).
- Emotional ESAS score: calculated as the sum of depression and anxiety symptoms (ranging from 0 to 20).
- The total ESAS score: calculated as the sum of all ten symptoms (ranging from 0 to 100).

2.3.3. Quality of Life

The European Organization for Research and Treatment of Cancer Quality of Life Questionnaire-Core 30 (EORTC QLQ-C30) score was developed to assess the quality of life of cancer patients. The EORTC QLQ-C30 questionnaire version 3.0 of this instrument includes 30 questions covering five functional domains (physical, role, cognitive, emotional, and social), eight symptoms (fatigue, nausea/vomiting, pain, dyspnoea, insomnia, loss of appetite, constipation, and diarrhea), and the financial impact produced by the disease. The questionnaire is scored on a four-point scale (ranging from 1 = "Not at all" to 4 = "A lot"), and these questions are scored from 0 to 100. In addition, general health and quality of life are rated on a seven-point scale ranging from 1 (="Very poor") to 7 (="Excellent"), with a score range of 0 to 100 representing the patient's overall health status, where 100 is the best possible condition [24]. High scores on the global health and functional scales indicate better quality of life, whereas on the symptom scale it would indicate decreased quality of life as it indicates the presence of cancer-related symptoms [24].

The validity and reliability of the Spanish version of the EORTC QLQ-C30 have been demonstrated as an effective tool for assessing quality of life in cancer patients. The reliability of the Spanish version of the questionnaire was found to be greater than 0.86, and the total score of the scale was a good indicator of the quality of life of cancer patients [25].

2.3.4. Satisfaction with the Health Care Received

This parameter was addressed using the Client Satisfaction Questionnaire-8 (CSQ-8), which includes eight Likert-scale questions rated from 1 to 4, resulting in a total score ranging from 8 to 32 points with higher scores indicating more satisfaction with the health care. Additionally, the questionnaire includes three open-ended questions asking patients to identify what they liked most and least about their health care, and what changes they would suggest [26].

The CSQ-8 is a brief, global index rating scale reliable in a variety of service settings to measure satisfaction with the health care received. Internal consistency reliability ranged from 0.83 to 0.90, supporting that the Spanish version of the questionnaire was reliable, valid, and linguistically equivalent to the English version [27].

2.4. Ethical Issues and Permissions

The study was granted ethical approval by the Malaga Provincial Ethics Committee, with project code 1752-N-18. All patients were informed about the study aims and methods both verbally and in writing. Signed informed consent to participate was requested and obtained from all participants. This project received funding support from the Regional Ministry for Health and Families in the field of primary care, through the Andalusian Health Service (SAS), under the project code AP-0157-2018. We took measures to protect the privacy and confidentiality of our participants, including the use of anonymized data and secure storage of personal information. We also disclosed any potential conflicts of interest, such as relationships with funding sources or commercial entities involved in the study, to ensure transparency and integrity in our research practices.

2.5. Data Collection

The patients were recruited to the study over a six-month period from January to December 2022. The final study sample was composed of 72 cancer patients receiving in-home palliative care, who met all the criteria for inclusion and who accepted the invitation to take part. A nurse subsequently visited these patients in their homes and asked them to complete the corresponding questionnaires.

2.6. Statistical Methods

The statistical data obtained are presented as mean ± standard deviation (SD) for the quantitative variables, and as absolute frequency (n) and percentage (%) for the categorical ones. Bivariate associations between the CSQ-8, EORTC QLQ-C30 and ESAS scores were analyzed using Spearman's nonparametric correlation test. Moreover, multiple linear regression was applied with the CSQ-8 as the predicted outcome and with EORTC QLQ-C30 and ESAS as independent variables. The SPSS 22 statistical software was used for all these analyses. Statistical significance was considered at a p-value of less than 0.05.

3. Results

3.1. Recruitment

Of the 78 patients initially assessed, three were excluded due to not meeting the eligibility criteria, two declined the invitation, and one passed away before the scheduled interview. The sociodemographic and clinical characteristics of the final sample (n = 72) are presented in Table 1.

Table 1. Sociodemographic and clinical characteristics of palliative cancer patients (n = 72).

Sociodemographic Variables	M	SD
Age (years)	74.61	10.13
	N	%
Gender		
Male	39	54.2
Female	33	45.8
Marital status		
Married	38	50.8
Widowed	23	31.9
Single	9	12.5
Divorced	2	2.8
Education level		
Primary education	29	40.3
No formal education	21	29.2
Secondary education	16	22.2
Higher education	6	8.3
Clinical variables	**M**	**SD**
Duration of palliative care (months)	4.88	5.84
	N	%
Type of cancer		
Colon	13	18.1
Lung	10	13.9
Breast	7	9.7
Pancreatic	6	8.3
Rectal	5	6.9
Prostate	4	5.6
Liver	4	5.6
Oropharyngeal	4	5.6
Kidney	4	5.6
Lymphoma	4	5.6
Bladder	3	4.2
Brain	3	4.2
Cervical	3	4.2
Ovarian	2	2.8

M: Mean, SD: Standard Deviation.

3.2. Study Variables

In our sample, the evaluation of the patients' symptoms is presented in Table 2. The mean of the total ESAS score of cancer patients was 32.25 ± 15.69 points, with a range from 0 to 100 points, where 0 is the best possible condition.

The perceived quality of life, based on the EORTC QLQ-C30 findings, is described in Table 3. The mean of the Global Health Status of cancer patients was 46.30 ± 23.27 points, with a range from 0 to 100 points, where 100 is the best possible condition.

Finally, descriptive results regarding the patients' satisfaction with health care assessed through the CSQ-8 are shown in Table 4. The mean total satisfaction score was 19.72 ± 3.34 points, with a range from 8 to 32 points, where 32 is the best possible condition.

Table 2. Results of the Edmonton Symptom Assessment System of 72 palliative cancer patients.

Symptoms (Range 0 to 10, 10 Being the Worst Possible Severity)	M	SD
Pain	4.31	3.12
Fatigue	5.79	2.64
Nausea	0.86	1.88
Depression	4.06	3.23
Anxiety	3.47	3.24
Drowsiness	3.90	3.10
Dyspnea	1.85	2.93
Loss of appetite	3.76	3.24
Reduced wellbeing	5.43	2.58
Sleep disorders	3.35	2.98
Classification of symptoms	**M**	**SD**
Physical (range 0 to 60, 60 being the worst possible severity)	20.61	10.39
Emotional (range 0 to 40, 40 being the worst possible severity)	7.53	5.94
Total ESAS symptoms (range 0 to 100, 100 being the worst possible severity)	32.25	15.69

ESAS: Edmonton Symptom Assessment System, M: Mean, SD: Standard Deviation.

Table 3. Self-reported quality of life assessed with the EORTC QLQ-C 30 in 72 cancer patients.

Scores from 0 to 100	M	SD
Global health status (100 indicates the best condition)	46.30	23.27
Functional scales (100 indicates the best condition)		
Physical functioning	60.65	32.80
Role functioning	61.57	34.22
Emotional functioning	39.51	25.80
Cognitive functioning	28.70	27.72
Social functioning	52.78	32.26
Symptom scales (0 indicates the best condition)		
Fatigue	52.16	24.27
Nausea/vomiting	5.56	16.55
Pain	45.60	33.10
Dyspnea	23.61	32.82
Insomnia	35.65	34.18
Loss of appetite	27.78	34.03
Constipation	9.72	22.68
Diarrhoea	7.45	21.10
Financial difficulties	17.50	26.14

EORTC QLQ-C 30: European Organization for Research and Treatment of Cancer Quality of Life Questionnaire-Core 30 version 3, M: Mean, SD: Standard Deviation.

Table 4. Results of the Client Satisfaction Questionnaire-8 in 72 in-home palliative cancer patients.

Items (Range 1 to 4, Where 4 Is the Best Condition)	M	SD
How would you rate the quality of service you received?	3.18	0.64
Did you get the kind of service you wanted?	2.06	0.71
To what extent has our service met your needs?	2.24	0.90
If a friend were in need of similar help, would you recommend our service to him or her?	2.00	0.75
How satisfied are you with the amount of help you received?	1.86	0.92
Have the services you received helped you to deal more effectively with your problems?	2.88	0.71
In an overall, general sense, how satisfied are you with the service you received?	3.43	0.67
If you were to seek help again, would you come back to our service?	2.08	0.85
Total score of the CSQ-8 (range 8 to 32, where 32 is the best condition)	19.72	3.34

CSQ-8: Client Satisfaction Questionnaire-8, M: Mean, SD: Standard Deviation.

3.3. Bivariate Associations and Regression Analysis

The bivariate relationships between the EORTC QLQ-C30 (Global Health Status), ESAS scale score, and CSQ-8 are presented in Table 5, and significant associations were found in all cases.

Table 5. Bivariate associations of satisfaction with health care, self-reported quality of life, and symptoms of 72 palliative cancer patients.

Spearman's Rho	CSQ-8	ESAS	EORTC QLQ-C30
CSQ-8	-	−0.397 *	0.486 *
ESAS	−0.296 *	-	−0.490 *
EORTC QLQ-C30	0.426 *	−0.490 *	-

* means $p < 0.05$. CSQ-8: Client Satisfaction Questionnaire-8, ESAS: Edmonton Symptom Assessment System, EORTC QLQ-C30: European Organisation for Research and Treatment of Cancer Quality of Life Questionnaire-Core 30 version 3.

The bivariate associations of the CSQ-8 with the level of ESAS symptoms showed that a higher satisfaction with the health care was significantly associated with lower severity of symptoms experienced by cancer patients (Spearman's rho = −0.397, $p = 0.001$).

The bivariate associations of the CSQ-8 with the Global Health Status assessed with the EORTC QLQ-C30 reported that the patients who presented higher satisfaction with their health care also demonstrated significantly higher levels of perceived Global Health Status ($r = 0.486$, $p < 0.001$).

Moreover, a higher quality of life (the EORTC QLQ-C30 total score) was associated with lower severity of symptoms assessed with the ESAS scale ($r = -0.511$, $p < 0.001$).

Using the CSQ-8 scale as the dependent variable, multiple linear regression analysis is presented in Table 6. An increment of 1 point on ESAS was related to a 0.5-point decrease of CSQ-8, while an increment of 1 point on EORTC QLQ-C30 was related to a 0.64-point increase in CSQ-8.

Table 6. Regression analysis of the CSQ-8 with quality of life and symptoms of 72 cancer patients.

	B	SE	p
Edmonton Symptom Assessment System	−0.504	0.017	0.001
EORTC QLQ-C30	−0.640	0.026	0.002

Dependent variable: CSQ-8, $R^2 = 0.338$, with $p < 0.001$. CSQ-8: Client Satisfaction Questionnaire-8, EORTC QLQ-C30: European Organisation for Research and Treatment of Cancer Quality of Life Questionnaire-Core 30 version 3.

4. Discussion

The study sample comprised of an equal proportion of men and women with an average age of 71 years. The most commonly observed types of cancer were colon, breast, and lung cancer, with frequencies of occurrence comparable to those reported in international studies [28]. The fact that the most commonly observed types of cancer in this study were consistent with those reported in international studies suggests that the study findings may be applicable to a broad range of patients with advanced cancer.

The mean duration of palliative treatment in our study can be considered acceptable, but earlier referral would be preferable. However, other studies have reported even shorter durations of palliative care, from referral until death [29]. It is now generally agreed that therapeutic and palliative care for cancer patients should be more closely integrated, as this could enhance the overall care received [2].

The ESAS results revealed that fatigue, reduced well-being, pain, drowsiness, and depression were the symptoms experienced with the highest intensity. These symptoms were previously identified in another study [30], although at a slightly higher severity level. In our sample, these symptoms were classified as having moderate severity (scores ranging from 4 to 6); nevertheless, the individual experience of each patient may vary [31,32]. A major barrier to adequate symptom treatment is poor assessment [33]. Symptom assessment is initiated with the use of standardized scales emphasizing anxiety, depression, physical symptoms, and coping strategies. These scales help to assess the severity of symptoms and guide symptom management. For effective palliative care, it is essential to use a standardized approach to symptom assessment that enables accurate identification of symptoms and their impact on patient's quality of life [5].

The average score for overall quality of life, as measured by the Global Health Status findings, among these patients with advanced cancer was >47 points, indicating a moderate-to-poor level of quality of life. This value is consistent with that found in comparable studies [34,35]. The finding that patients with advanced cancer in this study reported a moderate-to-poor level of quality of life highlights the importance of providing effective supportive care interventions to address symptoms and improve overall well-being. Given that this result is consistent with findings from comparable studies, it suggests that health care providers should prioritize interventions that have been shown to be effective in improving quality of life in this patient population. Additionally, the use of the Global Health Status measure provides a standardized tool for assessing quality of life in patients with advanced cancer, which can be useful for clinical decision-making and evaluating the effectiveness of interventions over time. Overall, these findings can inform the development and implementation of interventions aimed at improving quality of life for patients with advanced cancer.

On a scale of 8 to 32 points (where 32 represents the best possible condition), the patients' satisfaction with the healthcare they received was around 20 points. The item on the CSQ-8 survey that received the lowest score was related to "How satisfied are you with the amount of help you received?", highlighting the need for greater support for in-home palliative care. Out of all the items on the survey, only two ("How would you rate the quality of service you received?" and "In an overall, general sense, how satisfied are you with the service you received?") received a mean score higher than 3 points on a scale of 1 to 4. These findings suggest that there is room for improvement in patient satisfaction, as well as in the severity of the symptoms they experienced and their overall quality of life. The evaluation of satisfaction with care is a valuable approach for assessing the quality of cancer care. Satisfaction with care represents a significant domain in cancer outcomes research, although its full potential has yet to be explored [36].

Regarding the bivariate associations observed, it was found that more intense symptoms and lower quality of life are associated with lower satisfaction with health care received [36]. Similarly, when symptoms are more severe, the quality of life is lower. Conversely, patients who are most satisfied with the health care received usually experience less severe symptoms and have a better quality of life. The regression analysis showed that an increase of one point on the symptoms scale (assessed with ESAS) was associated with a decrease of half a point on the satisfaction scale (assessed with CSQ-8). Similarly, an increase of one point on the scale of quality of life (assessed with EORTC QLQ-C30) was associated with a slightly greater than half a point increase on the satisfaction scale.

These findings suggest that symptom control and improvement in quality of life are important factors in enhancing patient satisfaction with health care. While the relationship between patients' satisfaction with health care, quality of life, and symptom intensity may seem obvious, it is important to empirically demonstrate and quantify these associations to emphasize the significance of understanding patients' experiences in this regard.

A previous study [37] reported that, compared to usual oncology care, a concurrent nurse-led, palliative care-focused intervention addressing physical, psychosocial, and care coordination led to higher scores for quality of life and mood, but not to improvements in symptom intensity scores or reduced hospitalization or emergency department visits. Thus, the early integration of palliative care has been shown to enhance the quality of life and satisfaction with care and is now more widely recommended for patients with advanced cancer [38]. Providing early palliative care enhances satisfaction with care in advanced cancer by effectively addressing patients' emotional distress and quality of life, improving collaborative relationships with healthcare providers, and addressing concerns about end-of-life preparation [39]. Moreover, a recent study concluded that an early integration of palliative care is recommended for patients with advanced cancer, as it has been shown to both enhance quality of life and alleviate symptom burden [40].

Notwithstanding, a Cochrane review [41] suggested that there is low-quality evidence supporting that compared to usual care, specialist palliative care may provide small benefits for patient outcomes such as health-related quality of life, symptom burden, and patient satisfaction with care. Therefore, more well-conducted studies are needed to draw stronger conclusions and to assess the cost-effectiveness of this palliative care [41]. Terminal cancer patients require extensive and continuous care from health care professionals, but the causes of dissatisfaction and ways to improve it are not clear from the literature review [42], since it requires a comprehensive assessment of patients' satisfaction with care [43,44].

The present study finds that patients' dissatisfaction is associated with decreased quality of life and increased multiple symptoms among advanced cancer patients. This highlights the need for improved care for this patient population. Identifying the factors that contribute to the dissatisfaction of patients with terminal cancer can lead to the development of interventions and strategies that improve their quality of life and overall satisfaction with care. For instance, health care providers could focus on managing symptoms more effectively, improving communication and information-sharing with patients, and involving patients and their families in shared decision-making. Such improvements could ultimately lead to better patient outcomes and experiences.

5. Limitations

The present study is subject to the following limitations, and the results should be interpreted accordingly. Firstly, it is cross-sectional, and so the direction and causality of the effects recorded cannot be inferred. Additionally, information on the duration of time since the suspension of systemic treatment was not collected, which may have influenced the observed outcomes. Moreover, variables other than those studied may also influence patients' satisfaction with their health care. Hence, randomized controlled trials are encouraged to analyze the effect of interventions aimed at improving satisfaction with care and their relationship with quality of life and symptom severity in palliative care patients with cancer.

Furthermore, the sample size was limited, due to the relatively small number of cancer patients in our population receiving in-home palliative care. Although the present study is multicenter, involving six health centers in Andalusia, Spain, it may not be fully representative of the entire population of cancer patients receiving palliative care in other regions or countries. Therefore, the generalizability of the study findings may be limited. Additionally, cultural and socioeconomic differences between regions or countries may also influence patients' experiences and satisfaction with health care, which should be taken into consideration when interpreting the results of this study. Moreover, the study may be affected by selection bias, as patients who agreed to participate in the study may differ from those who declined or were unable to participate. Finally, self-reported symptoms may be subject to recall bias or individual interpretation.

6. Conclusions

The study shows that dissatisfaction among advanced cancer patients is linked to lower quality of life and increased symptoms, emphasizing the need for better care. Indeed, patients' satisfaction with the healthcare they received was around 20 points out of 32, indicating room for improvement in patient satisfaction and the severity of symptoms. The evaluation of satisfaction with care is important in assessing the quality of cancer care, and there is a need to explore its full potential for in-home palliative care.

The study found that fatigue, reduced well-being, pain, drowsiness, and depression were the most intense symptoms experienced by patients with moderate severity. Standardized scales are important in assessing the severity of symptoms and guiding symptom management and care. The use of the ESAS tool provides a standardized way to assess symptom intensity, which can aid in identifying patients who may require additional interventions and monitoring the effectiveness of interventions over time.

Moreover, the study's finding that patients with advanced cancer had a moderate-to-poor quality of life underscores the need for effective supportive care interventions. Given the consistency with similar studies, healthcare providers should prioritize proven interventions. The use of the standardized Global Health Status measure is useful for evaluating the effectiveness of interventions and guiding clinical decisions. These findings can inform the development of interventions aimed at improving quality of life for patients with advanced cancer.

When in-home palliative care is provided to patients with advanced cancer, it is important to determine their satisfaction with this process, together with their assessment of the symptoms presented. Both factors are relevant to the quality of health care and, ultimately, to the self-perceived quality of life. Identifying factors that contribute to dissatisfaction can lead to interventions that improve patient satisfaction, such as improving symptom management, communication with patients, and involving them in decision-making. Such improvements could lead to better patient outcomes and experiences.

In conclusion, these findings can be applied in practice by encouraging health care providers to routinely assess and address patient satisfaction during in-home palliative care. This may help to alleviate symptoms and improve quality of life for patients, while also providing them with emotional and social support during a difficult time. In addition, early referral to palliative care services can help to ensure that patients receive appropriate end-of-life care, such as advance care planning and symptom management, in a timely and compassionate manner. While the mean duration of palliative treatment in our study was considered acceptable, efforts to promote earlier referral to palliative care services may further improve the quality of care received by patients with advanced cancer.

Further research is necessary to identify effective interventions and establish a causal relationship between satisfaction with care and improved patient outcomes in the context of palliative care for cancer patients. These studies will help inform the development of evidence-based practices and policies for providing optimal palliative care to cancer patients in need.

Author Contributions: M.Á.V.-S. and C.C. contributed to the fundraising, conceptualization, methodological design, software application, formal analysis, background research, data curation, drafting, reviewing and editing of this study. I.V.-C. contributed to the fundraising, project management, conceptualization, methodological design, background research, review and editing. M.E.-T., F.J.B.-L. and F.J.M.-V. contributed to the conceptualization, methodological design, background research, review and editing. All authors have read and agreed to the published version of the manuscript.

Funding: External funding for this study, involving research, development, and innovation (R + D + I) in biomedical and health sciences in Andalusia (Spain), was obtained from the Regional Health Ministry of "Junta de Andalucia", under Project AP-0157-2018, dated 13 November 2018.

Institutional Review Board Statement: The study was conducted in accordance with the Declaration of Helsinki, and protocol was reviewed and approved by the Research Ethics Committee of the Province of Malaga, on 28 March 2019 (File number: AP-0157-2018).

Informed Consent Statement: Informed consent was obtained from all subjects involved in the study.

Data Availability Statement: Study data are available on reasonable request to the corresponding author.

Conflicts of Interest: The authors declare no conflict of interest.

References

1. Wild, C.P.; Weiderpass, E.; Stewart, B.W. *World Cancer Report: Cancer Research for Cancer Prevention*; World Cancer Reports; International Agency for Research on Cancer: Lyon, France, 2020.
2. Kaasa, S.; Loge, J.H.; Aapro, M.; Albreht, T.; Anderson, R.; Bruera, E.; Brunelli, C.; Caraceni, A.; Cervantes, A.; Currow, D.C.; et al. Integration of oncology and palliative care: A Lancet Oncology Commission. *Lancet Oncol.* **2018**, *19*, e588–e653. [CrossRef] [PubMed]
3. Lee, G.; Kim, H.S.; Lee, S.W.; Park, Y.R.; Kim, E.H.; Lee, B.; Hu, Y.J.; Kim, K.A.; Kim, D.; Cho, H.Y.; et al. Pre-screening of patient-reported symptoms using the Edmonton Symptom Assessment System in outpatient palliative cancer care. *Eur. J. Cancer Care* **2020**, *29*, e13305. [CrossRef] [PubMed]
4. Yates, P. Symptom Management and Palliative Care for Patients with Cancer. *Nurs. Clin. N. Am.* **2017**, *52*, 179–191. [CrossRef]
5. Hussaini, Q.; Smith, T.J. Incorporating palliative care into oncology practice: Why and how. *Clin. Adv. Hematol. Oncol.* **2021**, *19*, 390–395. [PubMed]
6. Nipp, R.D.; El-Jawahri, A.; Moran, S.M.; D'Arpino, S.M.; Johnson, P.C.; Lage, D.E.; Wong, R.L.; Pirl, W.F.; Traeger, L.; Lennes, I.T.; et al. The relationship between physical and psychological symptoms and health care utilization in hospitalized patients with advanced cancer. *Cancer* **2017**, *123*, 4720–4727. [CrossRef]
7. Miceli, J.; Geller, D.; Tsung, A.; Hecht, C.L.; Wang, Y.; Pathak, R.; Cheng, H.; Marsh, W.; Antoni, M.; Penedo, F.; et al. Illness perceptions and perceived stress in patients with advanced gastrointestinal cancer. *Psychooncology* **2019**, *28*, 1513–1519. [CrossRef] [PubMed]
8. Komarzynski, S.; Huang, Q.; Lévi, F.A.; Palesh, O.G.; Ulusakarya, A.; Bouchahda, M.; Haydar, M.; Wreglesworth, N.I.; Morère, J.-F.; Adam, R.; et al. The day after: Correlates of patient-reported outcomes with actigraphy-assessed sleep in cancer patients at home (inCASA project). *Sleep* **2019**, *42*, zsz146. [CrossRef]
9. Seow, H.; Stevens, T.; Barbera, L.C.; Burge, F.; McGrail, K.; Chan, K.K.W.; Peacock, S.J.; Sutradhar, R.; Guthrie, D.M. Trajectory of psychosocial symptoms among home care patients with cancer at end-of-life. *Psychooncology* **2021**, *30*, 103–110. [CrossRef]
10. Hui, D.; Bruera, E. The Edmonton Symptom Assessment System 25 Years Later: Past, Present, and Future Developments. *J. Pain Symptom Manag.* **2017**, *53*, 630–643. [CrossRef]
11. Chasen, M.; Bhargava, R.; Dalzell, C.; Pereira, J.L. Attitudes of oncologists towards palliative care and the Edmonton Symptom Assessment System (ESAS) at an Ontario cancer center in Canada. *Support. Care Cancer* **2015**, *23*, 769–778. [CrossRef]
12. Green, E.; Yuen, D.; Chasen, M.; Amernic, H.; Shabestari, O.; Brundage, M.; Krzyzanowska, M.; Klinger, C.; Ismail, Z.; Pereira, J. Oncology Nurses' Attitudes Toward the Edmonton Symptom Assessment System: Results from a Large Cancer Care Ontario Study. *Oncol. Nurs. Forum* **2017**, *44*, 116–125. [CrossRef] [PubMed]
13. Wong, A.; Tayjasanant, S.; Rodriguez-Nunez, A.; Park, M.; Liu, D.; Zapata, K.P.; Allo, J.; Frisbee-Hume, S.; Williams, J.; Bruera, E. Edmonton Symptom Assessment Scale Time Duration of Self-Completion Versus Assisted Completion in Patients with Advanced Cancer: A Randomized Comparison. *Oncologist* **2021**, *26*, 165–171. [CrossRef]
14. Borchert, K.; Jacob, C.; Wetzel, N.; Jänicke, M.; Eggers, E.; Sauer, A.; Marschner, N.; Altevers, J.; Mittendorf, T.; Greiner, W. Application study of the EQ-5D-5L in oncology: Linking self-reported quality of life of patients with advanced or metastatic colorectal cancer to clinical data from a German tumor registry. *Health Econ. Rev.* **2020**, *10*, 40. [CrossRef]
15. Kelly, M.; Rivas, C.; Foell, J.; Llewellyn-Dunn, J.; England, D.; Cocciadiferro, A.; Hull, S. Unmasking quality: Exploring meanings of health by doing art. *BMC Fam. Pract.* **2015**, *16*, 28. [CrossRef]
16. Diplock, B.D.; McGarragle, K.M.C.; Mueller, W.A.; Haddad, S.; Ehrlich, R.; Yoon, D.-H.A.; Cao, X.; Al-Allaq, Y.; Karanicolas, P.; Fitch, M.I.; et al. The impact of automated screening with Edmonton Symptom Assessment System (ESAS) on health-related quality of life, supportive care needs, and patient satisfaction with care in 268 ambulatory cancer patients. *Support. Care Cancer* **2019**, *27*, 209–218. [CrossRef]
17. Rietjens, J.A.C.; Sudore, R.L.; Connolly, M.; van Delden, J.J.; Drickamer, M.A.; Droger, M.; van der Heide, A.; Heyland, D.K.; Houttekier, D.; Janssen, D.J.A.; et al. Definition and recommendations for advance care planning: An international consensus supported by the European Association for Palliative Care. *Lancet Oncol.* **2017**, *18*, e543–e551. [CrossRef] [PubMed]
18. Jabbarian, L.J.; Zwakman, M.; Van Der Heide, A.; Kars, M.C.; Janssen, D.J.A.; Van Delden, J.J.; Rietjens, J.A.C.; Korfage, I.J. Advance care planning for patients with chronic respiratory diseases: A systematic review of preferences and practices. *Thorax* **2018**, *73*, 222–230. [CrossRef]
19. Zwakman, M.; Jabbarian, L.; van Delden, J.; van der Heide, A.; Korfage, I.; Pollock, K.; Rietjens, J.; Seymour, J.; Kars, M. Advance care planning: A systematic review about experiences of patients with a life-threatening or life-limiting illness. *Palliat. Med.* **2018**, *32*, 1305–1321. [CrossRef]
20. Lin, C.-P.; Evans, C.J.; Koffman, J.; Armes, J.; Murtagh, F.E.M.; Harding, R. The conceptual models and mechanisms of action that underpin advance care planning for cancer patients: A systematic review of randomised controlled trials. *Palliat. Med.* **2019**, *33*, 5–23. [CrossRef]
21. Korfage, I.J.; Carreras, G.; Christensen, C.M.A.; Billekens, P.; Bramley, L.; Briggs, L.; Bulli, F.; Caswell, G.; Červ, B.; Van Delden, J.J.M.; et al. Advance care planning in patients with advanced cancer: A 6-country, cluster-randomised clinical trial. *PLoS Med.* **2020**, *17*, e1003422. [CrossRef] [PubMed]
22. Bruera, E.; Kuehn, N.; Miller, M.J.; Selmser, P.; Macmillan, K. The Edmonton Symptom Assessment System (ESAS): A Simple Method for the Assessment of Palliative Care Patients. *J. Palliat. Care* **1991**, *7*, 6–9. [CrossRef] [PubMed]

23. Carvajal, A.; Centeno, C.; Watson, R.; Bruera, E. A comprehensive study of psychometric properties of the Edmonton Symptom Assessment System (ESAS) in Spanish advanced cancer patients. *Eur. J. Cancer* **2011**, *47*, 1863–1872. [CrossRef]
24. Aaronson, N.K.; Ahmedzai, S.; Bergman, B.; Bullinger, M.; Cull, A.; Duez, N.J.; Filiberti, A.; Flechtner, H.; Fleishman, S.B.; De Haes, J.C.J.M.; et al. The European Organization for Research and Treatment of Cancer QLQ-C30: A Quality-of-Life Instrument for Use in International Clinical Trials in Oncology. *JNCI J. Natl. Cancer Inst.* **1993**, *85*, 365–376. [CrossRef] [PubMed]
25. Calderon, C.; Ferrando, P.J.; Lorenzo-Seva, U.; Ferreira, E.; Lee, E.M.; Oporto-Alonso, M.; Obispo-Portero, B.M.; Mihic-Góngora, L.; Rodríguez-González, A.; Jiménez-Fonseca, P. Psychometric properties of the Spanish version of the European Organ-ization for Research and Treatment of Cancer Quality of Life Questionnaire (EORTC QLQ-C30). *Qual. Life Res.* **2022**, *31*, 1859–1869. [CrossRef] [PubMed]
26. Roberts, R.E.; Attkisson, C. Assessing client satisfaction among hispanics. *Eval. Program Plan.* **1983**, *6*, 401–413. [CrossRef] [PubMed]
27. Roberts, R.E.; Atrkisson, C.C.; Mendias, R.M. Assessing the Client Satisfaction Questionnaire in English and Spanish. *Hisp. J. Behav. Sci.* **1984**, *6*, 385–396. [CrossRef]
28. International Agency for Research on Cancer 2020. Data Source: Globocan 2018. Graph Production: Global Cancer Observa-Tory. Available online: http://gco.iarc.fr/ (accessed on 10 November 2022).
29. Bercow, A.S.; Nitecki, R.; Haber, H.; Gockley, A.A.; Hinchcliff, E.; James, K.; Melamed, A.; Diver, E.; Kamdar, M.M.; Feldman, S.; et al. Palliative care referral patterns and measures of aggressive care at the end of life in patients with cervical cancer. *Int. J. Gynecol. Cancer* **2021**, *31*, 66–72. [CrossRef]
30. Corli, O.; Pellegrini, G.; Bosetti, C.; Riva, L.; Crippa, M.; Amodio, E.; Scaccabarozzi, G. Impact of Palliative Care in Evaluating and Relieving Symptoms in Patients with Advanced Cancer. Results from the DEMETRA Study. *Int. J. Environ. Res. Public Health* **2020**, *17*, 8429. [CrossRef]
31. Seow, H.; Sussman, J.; Martelli-Reid, L.; Pond, G.; Bainbridge, D. Do High Symptom Scores Trigger Clinical Actions? An Audit After Implementing Electronic Symptom Screening. *J. Oncol. Pract.* **2012**, *8*, e142–e148. [CrossRef]
32. Hui, D.; Park, M.; Shamieh, O.; Paiva, C.E.; Perez-Cruz, P.E.; Muckaden, M.A.; Bruera, E. Personalized symptom goals and response in patients with advanced cancer. *Cancer* **2016**, *122*, 1774–1781. [CrossRef]
33. Cleeland, C.S. Cancer-related symptoms. *Semin. Radiat. Oncol.* **2000**, *10*, 175–190. [CrossRef]
34. Bjerring, O.S.; Larsen, M.K.; Fristrup, C.W.; Lundell, L.; Mortensen, M.B. The role of home visits by a nurse to improve palliation in patients treated with self-expandable metallic stents due to incurable esophageal cancer. *Dis. Esophagus* **2020**, *33*, doz076. [CrossRef] [PubMed]
35. Poort, H.; Peters, M.; van der Graaf, W.; Nieuwkerk, P.; van de Wouw, A.; der Sanden, M.N.-V.; Bleijenberg, G.; Verhagen, C.; Knoop, H. Cognitive behavioral therapy or graded exercise therapy compared with usual care for severe fatigue in patients with advanced cancer during treatment: A randomized controlled trial. *Ann. Oncol.* **2020**, *31*, 115–122. [CrossRef] [PubMed]
36. Jayadevappa, R.; Schwartz, J.S.; Chhatre, S.; Wein, A.J.; Malkowicz, S.B. Satisfaction with Care: A Measure of Quality of Care in Prostate Cancer Patients. *Med. Decis. Mak.* **2010**, *30*, 234–245. [CrossRef]
37. Bakitas, M.; Lyons, K.D.; Hegel, M.T.; Balan, S.; Brokaw, F.C.; Seville, J.; Hull, J.G.; Li, Z.; Tosteson, T.D.; Byock, I.R.; et al. Effects of a palliative care intervention on clinical outcomes in patients with advanced cancer: The Project ENABLE II randomized controlled trial. *JAMA* **2009**, *302*, 741–749. [CrossRef] [PubMed]
38. Hannon, B.; Swami, N.; Rodin, G.; Pope, A.; Zimmermann, C. Experiences of patients and caregivers with early palliative care: A qualitative study. *Palliat. Med.* **2017**, *31*, 72–81. [CrossRef] [PubMed]
39. Mah, K.; Swami, N.; O'Connor, B.; Hannon, B.; Rodin, G.; Zimmermann, C. Early palliative intervention: Effects on patient care satisfaction in advanced cancer. *BMJ Support. Palliat. Care* **2022**, *12*, 218–225. [CrossRef]
40. Kim, C.A.; Lelond, S.; Daeninck, P.J.; Rabbani, R.; Lix, L.; McClement, S.; Chochinov, H.M.; Goldenberg, B.A. The impact of early palliative care on the quality of life of patients with advanced pancreatic cancer: The IMPERATIVE case-crossover study. *Support. Care Cancer* **2023**, *31*, 250. [CrossRef]
41. Bajwah, S.; Oluyase, A.O.; Yi, D.; Gao, W.; Evans, C.J.; Grande, G.; Todd, C.; Costantini, M.; Murtagh, F.E.; Higginson, I.J. The effectiveness and cost-effectiveness of hospital-based specialist palliative care for adults with advanced illness and their caregivers. *Cochrane Database Syst. Rev.* **2020**, *2020*, CD012780. [CrossRef]
42. Carey, L.A.; Rugo, H.S.; Marcom, P.K.; Mayer, E.L.; Esteva, F.J.; Ma, C.X.; Liu, M.C.; Storniolo, A.M.; Rimawi, M.F.; Forero-Torres, A.; et al. TBCRC 001: Randomized Phase II Study of Cetuximab in Combination with Carboplatin in Stage IV Triple-Negative Breast Cancer. *J. Clin. Oncol.* **2012**, *30*, 2615–2623. [CrossRef] [PubMed]
43. Hall, A.; Bryant, J.; Sanson-Fisher, R.; Grady, A.; Proietto, A.; Doran, C.M. Top Priorities for Health Service Improvements Among Australian Oncology Patients. *Patient Relat. Outcome Meas.* **2021**, *12*, 83–95. [CrossRef] [PubMed]
44. Wang, T.; Molassiotis, A.; Chung, B.P.M.; Tan, J.-Y. Unmet care needs of advanced cancer patients and their informal caregivers: A systematic review. *BMC Palliat. Care* **2018**, *17*, 96. [CrossRef] [PubMed]

Disclaimer/Publisher's Note: The statements, opinions and data contained in all publications are solely those of the individual author(s) and contributor(s) and not of MDPI and/or the editor(s). MDPI and/or the editor(s) disclaim responsibility for any injury to people or property resulting from any ideas, methods, instructions or products referred to in the content.

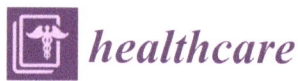

Article

Burden of Family Caregivers of Patients with Oral Cancer in Home Care in Taiwan

Tzu-Ting Chang [1], Shu-Yuan Liang [2,*] and John Rosenberg [3]

1. Department of Nursing, Taipei Veterans General Hospital, Taipei 112, Taiwan
2. School of Nursing, National Taipei University of Nursing and Health Sciences, Taipei 112, Taiwan
3. School of Health, University of the Sunshine Coast, Caboolture, QLD 4059, Australia
* Correspondence: shuyuan@ntunhs.edu.tw; Tel.: +886-2-28227101 (ext. 3105); Fax: +886-2-28213233

Abstract: Oral cancer is currently the fourth leading cause of cancer-related death in Taiwan. The complications and side effects of oral cancer treatment cause a tremendous burden on patients' family caregivers. This study explored the burden on primary family caregivers of patients with oral cancer and its related factors. One hundred and seven patients with oral cancer and their primary family caregivers were included through convenience sampling. The Caregiver Reaction Assessment (CRA) scale was employed as the primary research instrument. The primary factors of caregiver burden, in descending order, were disrupted schedules (M = 3.19, SD = 0.84), a lack of family support (M = 2.82, SD = 0.85), health problems (M = 2.67, SD = 0.68), and financial problems (M = 2.59, SD = 0.84). The CRA scores of the caregivers differed significantly in terms of education level (t = 2.57, $p < 0.05$) and household income (F = 4.62, $p < 0.05$), which significantly predicted caregiver burden ($R^2 = 0.11$, F = 4.32, $p = 0.007$). The study results provide a reference for healthcare professionals to identify the factors for family caregiver burden, as well as the characteristics of patients and family caregivers particularly vulnerable to caregiver burden, thus improving family-centred care.

Keywords: burden; family caregiver; oral cancer

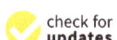

Citation: Chang, T.-T.; Liang, S.-Y.; Rosenberg, J. Burden of Family Caregivers of Patients with Oral Cancer in Home Care in Taiwan. Healthcare 2023, 11, 1107. https://doi.org/10.3390/healthcare11081107

Academic Editor: Qiuping Li

Received: 15 March 2023
Revised: 7 April 2023
Accepted: 11 April 2023
Published: 12 April 2023

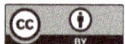

Copyright: © 2023 by the authors. Licensee MDPI, Basel, Switzerland. This article is an open access article distributed under the terms and conditions of the Creative Commons Attribution (CC BY) license (https://creativecommons.org/licenses/by/4.0/).

1. Introduction

In Taiwan, oral cancer is associated with alcohol and betel nut consumption [1,2]. More than 90% of the patients who have died of oral cancer in Taiwan have been men; oral cancer is the fourth most prominent cause of cancer-related death among men [3]. The complications, side effects, and risks of death associated with oral cancer treatment present a tremendous burden to the patients, patient families, and medical professionals in care provision.

Although oral cancer can be treated through a combination of surgery, chemotherapy, and radiotherapy, surgery is the main treatment of choice [4]. However, surgery alters the tissue structures of patients' mouths, faces, and jawbones, thus altering their facial appearances, chewing and swallowing functions, and communication abilities, in addition to causing pain [5–8]. Furthermore, patients are burdened by the side effects of chemotherapy and radiotherapy. Therefore, challenges in caregiving to patients with oral cancer can be greater than those in caregiving to patients with other types of cancer.

Families play a major role in caregiving to patients with oral cancer in Taiwan; families are required to provide direct home care and economic, social, and emotional support [9]. This challenging caregiving process causes a great burden on the time, finances, and health of these families [9]. It also causes fatigue and emotional effects on the caregiving families, severely affecting their physical and psychological health in the process [10]. Consequently, this can reduce the effectiveness of families' care for patients with oral cancer [11]. Studies report not all family caregivers of patients with oral cancer have negative experiences. Some family caregivers report positive experiences in caregiving to patients with oral cancer in terms of discovering the importance of caregiving for their family members with oral cancer and feeling an enhanced sense of dignity [12–15]. Some factors, however, such as the sociodemographic variables of patients and their families and the patient's medical condition, may exacerbate the caregiver burden.

Studies indicate a correlation between caregiver burden and age, sex, education level, marital status, religious affiliation, employment status, financial status, relationship with patients, whether they live with patients, length of care for patients, and whether they are supported by other family members [15–20]. Studies also report the possibility of a correlation between caregiver burden and patients' age, education level, religious affiliation, history of chronic diseases along with the disease stages, and type of treatment [15,17–19].

The study of the burden of primary family caregivers to patients with oral cancer and its related factors will help medical professionals to more clearly understand the caregiver burden status and, accordingly, provide family-centred care. The present study explored the burden of primary family caregivers in providing home care to patients with oral cancer and its related factors.

2. Methods

2.1. Study Design, Sample, and Procedure

A cross-sectional descriptive study was conducted, with convenience sampling. A structured questionnaire was administered from May 2016 to May 2018 to 107 outpatients with oral cancer from the radiology department in a teaching hospital in Northern Taiwan and their primary family caregivers. The inclusion criteria for the patients were (1) age 20 years or older, (2) diagnosis of oral cancer, and (3) receipt of surgery, chemotherapy, or radiotherapy targeting oral cancer. The inclusion criteria for the patients' primary family caregivers were as follows: (1) age 20 years or older, (2) primary family caregivers as recognised by the patients, and (3) living together with the patients. The exclusion criteria for primary caregiver were the primary caregiver had an employment relationship with the patient. This study was approved by the institutional review board of the hospital, and informed consent forms were signed by the patients and their primary family caregivers. The questionnaires were distributed by the research assistants and voluntarily filled in by the caregivers, after which the research assistants examined the responses on-site to check for any unanswered items. The family caregivers were requested by the assistants to fill in any items that were not answered. The patients' medical characteristics were collected from their medical history by the research assistants.

2.2. Ethical Considerations

This study was approved by the institutional review board of a teaching hospital (VGHIRB no.: 2014-04-001AC) in Northern Taiwan. The research assistants verbally explained the research objective, data protection method, and research procedure to the participants before acquiring signed consent from the participants. The participants' personal information was coded in the questionnaire to protect their privacy. Participants who were unwilling to continue being surveyed or unfit for further survey because of poor physical condition were free to withdraw from the study, and their data collection was discontinued by the researchers.

2.3. Measures

Sociodemographic Variables

The data collected in this study were the sociodemographic variables of the patients and their primary family caregivers, as well as the types of care and the patients' medical characteristics. The sociodemographic variables included sex, age, marital status, education level, religious affiliation, employment status, and household income. The medical characteristics included the time of oral cancer diagnosis, the stage of cancer, current treatment status, and reported side effects from the treatment. The data on the primary family caregivers also included their relationship with the patients and the type and length of care.

2.4. Caregiver Reaction Assessment

Caregiver Reaction Assessment (CRA), a tool used to assess caregiver burden, consists of 5 subscales encompassing 24 items, namely, disrupted schedules (5 items), financial problems (3 items), health problems (4 items), lack of family support (5 items), and self-esteem (7 items). While disrupted schedules, financial problems, health problems, and lack of family support constituted negative caregiver reactions, self-esteem constituted positive caregiver reactions. A 5-point Likert scale was employed (1 = strongly disagree; 5 = strongly agree), with a higher score indicating a higher caregiver burden [21]. The Cronbach's α of each subscale ranged between 0.68 and 0.90 [22,23]. According to the test–retest reliability test results, the intraclass correlation of the Chinese language edition of the scale was ≥ 0.75, and the edition exhibited sufficient construct validity [24]. The Cronbach's α of each subscale in this edition ranged between 0.70 and 0.92, and the total Cronbach's α of the edition was 0.82 [20].

2.5. Statistical Analysis

SPSS 22.0 for Windows was employed for statistical data analysis. Descriptive statistical analysis was performed on the means, standard deviations, frequencies, and percentages for the sociodemographic variables of all the participants, the patients' medical characteristics, the relationship between the primary family caregivers and the patients, the type and length of care, and caregiver burden (according to the CRA). The differences in caregiver burden based on various sociodemographic variables and medical characteristics were examined using analysis of variance and an independent sample *t*-test. The correlation between the CRA scores and the caregivers' and patients' age, length of patient care, and length of patient illness was analysed through Pearson product–moment correlation. Subsequently, multiple regression analysis was conducted on the caregiver burden predictive power of the sociodemographic variables and medical characteristics.

When certain sociodemographic variables and medical characteristics were significantly correlated with caregiver burden, dummy coding was to be conducted for the variables and characteristics that are discrete or nominal before conducting multiple regression analysis. During the multiple regression analysis, the sociodemographic variables, medical characteristics, the relationships between the primary family caregivers of the patients, and the types and lengths of care that are significantly correlated with caregiver burden were treated as independent predictors of caregiver burden, which is the dependent variable.

3. Results

3.1. Sociodemographic Variables of the Primary Family Caregivers

Of the 107 primary family caregivers, 98 were women (91.6%). The average age of these caregivers was 51 ± 10.8 years, and their ages ranged from 20 to 70 years. Regarding the relationships between the caregivers and patients, 78 of the caregivers were spouses to the patients (72.9%). Of these caregivers, 60 had senior high school or higher levels of education (56.1%); 94 were married (87.9%); 28 were employed and provided care to their patients after work (26.2%); 51 had household incomes of no higher than NT$500,000 (47.7%); 93 had religious affiliations (86.9%); and 28 were diagnosed with chronic diseases themselves (26.2%; Table 1).

Table 1. Differences in total burden of the primary family caregivers according to their sociodemographic variables and the type of care ($n = 107$).

Variable	Number	%	Mean	SD	t/F	p
Sex					t = 0.83	0.41
Male	9	8.4	2.87	0.29		
Female	98	91.6	2.72	0.53		
Relationship with patient					t = 1.19	0.24
Spouse	78	72.9	2.77	0.48		
Other	29	27.1	2.64	0.60		
Education level					t = 2.57 *	0.02
Junior high school or lower	47	43.9	2.87	0.40		
Senior high school or higher	60	56.1	2.63	0.57		
Marital status					t = 1.88	0.06
Married/cohabiting	94	87.9	2.77	0.49		
Other	13	12.1	2.49	0.63		
Employment status					F = 0.62	0.60
Quit their job	19	17.8	2.86	0.49		
Employed and providing care after work	28	26.2	2.65	0.55		
Employed but on leave	11	10.3	2.78	0.43		
Other	49	45.8	2.73	0.53		
Household income					F = 4.62 *	0.01
① ≤NT$500,000	51	47.7	2.89	0.49	① > ②	
② NT$510,000–NT$1,000,000	39	36.4	2.59	0.52		
③ ≥NT$1,010,000	17	15.9	2.62	0.47		
Religious affiliation					t = 0.71	0.49
Yes	93	86.9	2.76	0.48		
No	14	13.1	2.62	0.71		
Chronic disease					t = 0.07	0.94
Yes	28	26.2	2.73	0.43		
No	79	73.8	2.74	0.54		
Type of care					F = 2.75	0.07
Together with someone else	44	41.1	2.68	0.52		
Independent care throughout the day	28	26.2	2.93	0.36		
Independent care without provision throughout the day	35	32.7	2.66	0.58		
Length of care per week					F = 1.79	0.17
No rest	43	40.2	2.85	0.39		
Rest each week	24	22.4	2.63	0.51		
Irregular rest	40	37.4	2.68	0.61		
Patient care experience					t = −1.17	0.25
Yes	18	16.8	2.87	0.63		
No	89	83.2	2.71	0.49		

* $p < 0.05$. Total burden is calculated with self-esteem scored in reverse; a higher score indicates higher burden.

3.2. Types of Care Provided by the Primary Family Caregivers

Of the primary family caregivers, 44 provided care to their patients together with other family members or hired caregivers (41.1%), whereas 28 had to care for their patients independently throughout the day (26.2%). The primary family caregivers had provided care to their patients for an average of 36.4 ± 40.3 months, with the length of care ranging from 1 to 171 months. Of the caregivers, 43 had provided full care for patients each week (40.2%); 40 had irregular rest time each week (37.4%); and 89 were inexperienced in providing care to patients (83.20%; Table 1).

3.3. Sociodemographic Variables of the Patients

Of the 107 patients with oral cancer, 100 were men (93.5%), and the average age was 56.4 ± 9.7 years (range, 33–89 years). Of the total patients, 59 graduated from educational institutes no higher than junior high schools (55.1%); 38 remained employed in full-time jobs even after developing oral cancer (35.5%), but 37 were unemployed (34.6%); 88 lived with their families or friends (82.2%); and 87 had a religious affiliation (87.3%; Table 2).

Table 2. Differences in total burden according to patients' sociodemographic information and medical characteristics ($n = 107$).

Variable	Number	%	Mean	SD	t/F	p
Sex					$t = 1.43$	1.56
Male	100	93.5	2.76	0.51		
Female	7	6.5	2.47	0.50		
Education level					$t = -1.23$	0.22
Junior high school or lower	59	55.1	2.68	0.61		
Senior high school or higher	48	44.9	2.80	0.36		
Employment status					$F = 1.30$	0.28
Unemployed	37	34.5	2.87	0.54		
Full-time	38	35.5	2.67	0.50		
Retired	16	15.0	2.70	0.44		
Other	16	15	2.62	0.54		
Living with family or friends					$t = 0.50$	0.62
Yes	88	82.2	2.75	0.54		
No	19	17.8	2.68	0.39		
Religious affiliation					$t = -0.29$	0.78
Yes	87	87.3	2.74	0.48		
No	20	18.7	2.71	0.64		
Stage of cancer					$F = 0.97$	0.41
Stage 1	22	20.6	2.62	0.52		
Stage 2	32	29.9	2.71	0.62		
Stage 3	14	13.1	2.70	0.50		
Stage 4	39	36.4	2.84	0.41		
Received treatment					$t = 0.54$	0.59
Yes	23	21.5	2.69	0.63		
No	84	78.5	2.75	0.48		
Side effects from treatment					$t = 0.41$	0.68
Yes	39	36.4	2.71	0.54		
No	68	63.6	2.75	0.50		

Total burden is calculated with self-esteem scored in reverse; a higher score indicates higher burden.

3.4. Medical Characteristics

The patients had experienced oral cancer for 1–171 months, with an average of 42.5 ± 44.4 months. Of all the patients, 39 were at the fourth stage of oral cancer (36.4%), and 32 were at the second stage (29.9%); 84 had completed their treatment (78.5%); and 39 experienced the side effects of their treatment (36.4%; Table 2).

3.5. Caregiver Burden

CRA was used to assess the caregiver burden. Specifically, the assessment subscales were disrupted schedules, financial problems, health problems, a lack of family support, and self-esteem. The results reveal the highest average scores in disrupted schedules (3.19 ± 0.84), followed by a lack of family support (2.82 ± 0.85), health problems (2.67 ± 0.68), and financial problems (2.59 ± 0.84) among primary family caregivers to patients with oral cancer. However, the caregivers' feelings about providing care to their family members were not always negative. The caregivers obtained an average score of 3.58 ± 0.49 in self-esteem (Table 3). Thereafter, the self-esteem was scored in reverse, and the total average caregiver burden score was calculated; a higher total average score indicates a higher caregiver burden. The total average score was calculated as 2.74 ± 0.52, with the total score of each caregiver ranging from 1.31 to 3.87.

Table 3. Caregiver burden ($n = 107$).

Variable	Mean	SD	Minimum	Maximum
Disrupted schedule	3.19	0.84	1.20	5.00
Financial problem	2.59	0.84	1.00	4.60
Lack of family support	2.82	0.85	1.00	5.00
Health problem	2.67	0.68	1.00	4.50
Self-esteem	3.58	0.49	2.43	4.57

Higher scores indicate a higher burden, with the exception of scores in self-esteem, where a higher score indicates a lower burden.

3.6. Differences in the Burden of the Primary Family Caregivers According to Their Sociodemographic Variables and Type of Care

After self-esteem was scored in reverse, the total average score of the burden of the primary family caregivers was calculated; a higher score indicates a higher caregiver burden. The association of the sociodemographic variables and type of care with total burden was then investigated. The age of the caregivers ($r = 0.12$, $p > 0.05$) and the length of care ($r = 0.07$, $p > 0.05$) were not significantly correlated with the total average burden. Only the education level ($t = 2.57$, $p < 0.05$) and the household income ($F = 4.62$, $p < 0.05$) of the caregivers were significantly correlated with the total average burden, but no other sociodemographic variables and no type of care were significantly correlated with the total burden (Table 1).

3.7. Differences in Caregiver Burden According to Patients' Sociodemographic Variables and Medical Characteristics

The age of the patients ($r = 0.04$, $p > 0.05$) and the length of illness ($r = 0.09$, $p > 0.05$) were not significantly correlated with caregiver burden. Furthermore, the other sociodemographic variables and medical characteristics were not significantly correlated with the caregiver burden (Table 2).

3.8. Predictive Power of Sociodemographic Variables, Medical Characteristics, and Type of Care on Caregiver Burden

The education level and household income of the primary family caregivers were significantly correlated with the total burden. These variables were further analysed for their power of predicting caregiver burden through multiple regression. The collinearity tolerance values ranged between 0.44 and 0.92 (higher than the cut-off value of 0.10), and the variance inflation factors ranged between 1.09 and 2.26 (lower than the cut-off value of 10), indicating that the variables exhibited no collinearity [25]. In the multiple regression analysis, the education level and household income of the primary family caregivers were analysed through the enter approach and selected as the predictor variables for the total caregiver burden. These predictor variables significantly predicted the total variance of the caregivers' burden (11%; $p = 0.007$) (Table 4).

Table 4. Multiple Regression Analysis for Variables Predicting Family Caregiver Burden ($n = 107$).

Variable	B	SE B	β
Caregivers' education levels			
Senior high school or higher vs. junior high school or lower	−0.19	0.10	−0.18
Household income/year (NTD)			
≤NT$500,000 vs. ≥NT$1,010,000	0.20	0.14	0.19
NT$510,000–NT$1,000,000 vs. ≥NT$1,010,000	−0.07	0.15	−0.07
Overall model	$R^2 = 0.11$ ($F (3, 103) = 4.32$, $p = 0.007$)		

NTD—New Taiwan Dollar.

4. Discussion

This study examined the burden on primary family caregivers to patients with oral cancer and its related factors. The results may help medical professionals to understand the current status regarding caregiver burden and identify the family and patient characteristics that incur caregiver burden, facilitating family-centred care. The results of this study reveal that the primary family caregivers exhibited high self-esteem; disrupted schedules represented the most prominent factor to their burden, followed by a lack of family support, health problems, and financial problems.

Disrupted schedules were reported by the primary family caregivers as the greatest contributing factor to their burden, which is consistent with the findings of studies on the burden on primary family caregivers to patients with rectal, lung, oral, and terminal cancer [9,12–15,17,18,20]. In this study, nearly all the primary family caregivers were wives of the patients with oral cancer. Based on the findings regarding employment status and age, most caregivers were required to manage their jobs and take care of their young children in addition to providing care to the patients.

A lack of family support constituted the second most prominent factor to caregiver burden. This differs from the findings of most studies, which have indicated that a lack of family support is the least prominent contributor to caregiver burden [9,12–15,17,18,20]. In this study, only one-fourth of the caregivers provided care independently throughout the day; most of the caregivers provided care with the help of other people or provided care independently but not throughout the day. However, the helpers may not be members of the caregivers' families but caregivers hired from other countries, which may have caused the primary family caregivers to perceive family support as lacking. Supportive communication between family members is critical [26].

Health problems were the third highest contributor to caregiver burden, which is consistent with the findings in some of the existing studies [9,12,13,17]. Approximately one-fourth of the caregivers were themselves diagnosed as having chronic diseases, and most of the caregivers had received help from other people in providing care. Although health problems were only the third highest factor for caregiver burden, family caregivers experienced emotional stress in addition to physical fatigue in providing care to patients; this affects the caregivers' overall psychological health [27].

Many studies have indicated financial problems as the second greatest contributor to caregiver burden [9,12,13,17], but this study revealed it as the least prominent factor. In Taiwan, national health insurance covers the health care costs of the population in Taiwan, and patients with cancer are provided additional subsidies related to major diseases. Therefore, problems related to medical expenses may not be the primary factor for the burden of primary family caregivers. Nevertheless, the financial conditions of the caregivers' families contribute to the caregiver burden. Specifically, the caregivers with the lowest household incomes exhibited significantly heavier total burdens than the other caregivers.

In fact, household incomes significantly predict the overall burden of primary family caregivers. According to Cheng et al. [27], family caregivers of patients with oral cancer are required to deal with the treatment side effects. For example, patients may require nasogastric tube feeding or emergency treatment, which involves additional expenses. Occasionally, an additional cost is required to hire replacement caregivers. In Taiwan, oral cancer is primarily associated with betelnut consumption [1,2], and most betelnut consumers are working-class people with disadvantaged household economic conditions. Moreover, families may sometimes be required to resign from their jobs to take care of patients, further worsening their financial conditions. According to Cheng et al. [27], acquiring financial support is a critical problem faced by primary family caregivers. Therefore, financial problems remain a critical problem to these caregivers. Patients in Taiwan are included in the national health insurance system, so the financial problem is not the primary burden in the current population. However, according to the statistical results of the current study, financial status is a crucial variable that can significantly predict the burden of a family. Financial problems may still play an important role in the family burden for other populations not covered by health insurance.

The primary family caregivers scored high in self-esteem. Because self-esteem is a positive aspect of caregiver reactions, a higher score in self-esteem indicates a lower caregiver burden. This is consistent with the findings of most studies [9,12–15], indicating that the caregivers were willing to care for their family members who were ill and considered the task critical despite the huge burden it caused.

After self-esteem was scored in reverse, the total average caregiver burden score was calculated. A higher score indicates a higher total caregiver burden. The results of this study reveal that the education levels and household incomes of the primary family caregivers significantly predicted their total burden. The caregivers with higher education levels exhibited lower burdens than those with lower education levels, whereas those with lower household incomes experienced higher burdens than those with higher household incomes. Studies have reported that financial and educational problems in a family critically affect the caregiver burden [20,28,29]. Accordingly, medical professionals should pay utmost attention to family caregivers with low incomes or education levels and understand their needs in providing care.

A meta-analysis has shown that case management, psychoeducation, and multicomponent interventions can significantly reduce the burden on caregivers. In particular, case management and counselling appeared to be better than cognitive behavioural therapy [30]. The multiple components of REACH II intervention focused on social support, communication, selfcare, emotional well-being, and community support [31–33], which included access to support groups by videophone [33–35]. A case management program is specifically their adaptability and flexibility, which provides caregivers with the ability to respond to the complex needs of the family member they care for [36].

This study was a cross-sectional descriptive study and did not clarify the changes in the burden of primary family caregivers over changes in patients' conditions or time. Moreover, because participants were enrolled from only one teaching hospital in Northern Taiwan, the results may not be representative of all primary family caregivers. Convenience sampling used in the current study may cause sampling bias. Families with high care burdens may be eliminated inherently. On the other hand, the sample size was small for several sociodemographic and medical variable groups. It is unlikely that statistical differences could be detected in caregiver burden by patients' sociodemographic information and medical characteristics.

5. Conclusions

The primary factors contributing to the burden of primary family caregivers, in descending order, were disrupted schedules, a lack of family support, health problems, and financial problems. The results of this study reveal that the caregivers exhibited high self-esteem, which is a positive aspect of caregiver reactions. Although home care presented a huge burden to the primary family caregivers, the caregivers were still willing to provide care and considered it pivotal. Moreover, low household income and low education levels significantly affected the caregiver burden.

Medical professionals should prioritise the arrangement of primary family caregivers' time for care in their education strategies. Referral of related care resources is also crucial in providing family caregivers adequate time to rest. Additionally, supportive communication between family members must be promoted. Self-care strategies should be taught to family caregivers. Furthermore, economically disadvantaged families, particularly those with low education levels, should be assisted in finding substantial support from social welfare institutions.

This study recommends that future research builds on the results of this current study and focuses on the development of relevant interventions to reduce the burden of primary caregivers at home.

Author Contributions: Conceptualization and methodology, T.-T.C. and S.-Y.L.; investigation, T.-T.C.; data curation, S.-Y.L.; formal analysis, S.-Y.L.; writing—original draft preparation, S.-Y.L.; writing—review and editing, J.R.; supervision and project administration, S.-Y.L. All authors have read and agreed to the published version of the manuscript.

Funding: This research received no external funding.

Institutional Review Board Statement: The study was conducted in accordance with the Declaration of Helsinki, and approved by the Institutional Review Board of TAIPEI VETERANS GENERAL HOSPITAL (protocol code: 2014-04-001 AC; date of approval: 5 May 2014).

Informed Consent Statement: Informed consent was obtained from all subjects involved in the study.

Data Availability Statement: The data presented in this study are available from the corresponding author upon reasonable request.

Conflicts of Interest: The authors declare no conflict of interest.

References

1. Ho, P.S.; Ko, Y.C.; Yang, Y.H.; Shieh, T.Y.; Tsai, C.C. The incidence of oropharyngeal cancer in Taiwan: An endemic betel quid chewing area. *J. Oral. Pathol. Med.* **2002**, *31*, 213–219. [CrossRef]
2. Tsou, H.H.; Hu, C.H.; Liu, J.H.; Liu, C.J.; Lee, C.H.; Liu, T.Y.; Wang, H.T. Acrolein is involved in the synergistic potential of cigarette smoking- and betel quid chewing-related human oral cancer. *Cancer Epidemiol Biomark. Prev.* **2019**, *28*, 954–962. [CrossRef]
3. Ministry of Health and Welfare Cancer Registry Annual Report. 2018. Available online: https://www.hpa.gov.tw/Pages/Detail.aspx?nodeid=269&pid=13498 (accessed on 10 October 2021).
4. Lin, M.C.; Leu, Y.S.; Chiang, C.J.; Ko, J.Y.; Wang, C.P.; Yang, T.L.; Chen, T.C.; Chen, C.N.; Chen, H.L.; Liao, C.T.; et al. Adequate surgical margins for oral cancer: A Taiwan cancer registry national database analysis. *Oral Oncol.* **2021**, *119*, 105358. [CrossRef]
5. Gobbo, M.; Bullo, F.; Perinetti, G.; Gatto, A.; Ottaviani, G.; Biasotto, M.; Tirelli, G. Diagnostic and therapeutic features associated with modification of quality-of-life's outcomes between one and six months after major surgery for head and neck cancer. *Braz J Otorhinolaryngol.* **2016**, *82*, 548–557. [CrossRef]
6. Semple, C.J.; Dunwoody, L.; Kernohan, W.G. Changes and challenges to patients' lifestyle patterns following treatment for head and neck cancer. *J. Adv. Nurs.* **2008**, *63*, 85–93. [CrossRef]
7. Ronis, D.L.; Duffy, S.A.; Fowler, K.E.; Khan, M.J.; Terrell, J.E. Changes in quality of life over 1 year in patients with head and neck cancer. *Arch. Otolaryngol. Head Neck Surg.* **2008**, *134*, 241–248. [CrossRef]
8. Trzcieniecka-Green, A.; Bargiel-Matusiewicz, K.; Borczyk, J. Quality of life of patients after laryngectomy. *J. Physiol. Pharmacol.* **2007**, *58*, 699–704.
9. Chen, S.C.; Tsai, M.C.; Liu, C.L.; Yu, W.P.; Liao, C.T.; Chang, J.T.C. Support needs of patients with oral cancer and burden to their family caregivers. *Cancer Nurs.* **2009**, *32*, 473–481. [CrossRef]
10. Johansen, S.; Cvancarova, M.; Ruland, C. The effect of cancer patients' and their family caregivers' physical and emotional symptoms on caregiver burden. *Cancer Nurs.* **2018**, *41*, 91–99. [CrossRef]
11. Baker, A.; Barker, S.; Sampson, A.; Martin, C. Caregiver outcomes and interventions: A systematic scoping review of the traumatic brain injury and spinal cord injury literature. *Clin. Rehabil.* **2017**, *31*, 45–61. [CrossRef] [PubMed]
12. Hanly, P.; Maguire, R.; Hyland, P.; Sharp, L. Examining the role of subjective and objective burden in carer health-related quality of life: The case of colorectal cancer. *Support. Care Cancer* **2015**, *23*, 1941–1949. [CrossRef]
13. Milbury, K.; Badr, H.; Fossella, F.; Pisters, K.M.; Carmack, C.L. Longitudinal associations between caregiver burden and patient and spouse distress in couples coping with lung cancer. *Support. Care Cancer* **2013**, *21*, 2371–2379. [CrossRef]
14. Shieh, S.C.; Tung, H.H.; Liang, S.Y. Social support as influencing primary family caregiver burden in Taiwanese patients with colorectal cancer. *J. Nurs. Scholarsh.* **2012**, *44*, 223–231. [CrossRef]
15. Utne, I.; Miaskowski, C.; Paul, S.M.; Rustøen, T. Association between hope and burden reported by family caregivers of patients with advanced cancer. *Support. Care Cancer* **2013**, *21*, 2527–2535. [CrossRef]
16. Francis, L.E.; Worthington, J.; Kypriotakis, G.; Rose, J.H. Relationship quality and burden among caregivers for late-stage cancer patients. *Support. Care Cancer* **2010**, *18*, 429–1436. [CrossRef]
17. Maguire, P.; Hanly, P.; Hyland, P.; Sharp, L. Understanding burden in caregivers of colorectal cancer survivors: What role do patient and caregiver factors play? *Eur. J. Cancer Care* **2018**, *27*, e12527. [CrossRef]
18. Park, C.H.; Shin, D.W.; Choi, J.Y.; Kang, J.; Baek, Y.J.; Mo, H.N.; Lee, M.S.; Park, S.J.; Park, S.M.; Park, S. Determinants of the burden and positivity of family caregivers of terminally ill cancer patients in Korea. *Psycho-Oncol.* **2012**, *21*, 282–290.
19. Ramli, S.F.; Pardi, K.W. Factors associated with caregiver burden of family with a cancer patient undergoing chemotherapy at a tertiary hospital, Malaysia. *Int. Med. J.* **2018**, *25*, 99–102.
20. Wong, C.L.; Choi, K.C.; Lau, M.N.; Lam, K.L.; So, W.K.W. Caregiving burden and sleep quality amongst family caregivers of Chinese male patients with advanced cancer: A cross-sectional study. *Eur. J. Oncol. Nurs.* **2020**, *46*, 101774. [CrossRef]

21. Nijboer, C.; Triemstra, M.; Tempelaar, R.; Sanderman, R.; Bos, G. Detrminants of caregiving experiences and mental health of partners of cancer patients. *Cancer* **1999**, *86*, 577–588.
22. Given, C.W.; Given, B.; Stommel, M.; Collins, C.; King, S.; Franklin, S. The Caregiver Reaction Assessment (CRA) for Caregivers to Persons with Chronic Physical and Mental Impairments. *Res. Nurs. Health* **1992**, *15*, 271–283. [CrossRef]
23. Nijboer, C.; Triemstra, M.; Tempelaar, R.; Sanderman, R.; Bos, G. Measuring both negative and positive reactions to giving care to cancer patients: Psychometric qualities of the Caregiver Reaction Assessment (CRA). *Soc. Sci. Med.* **1999**, *48*, 1259–1269. [CrossRef]
24. Ge, C.; Yang, X.; Fu, J.; Chang, Y.; Wei, J.; Zhang, F.; Nutifafa, A.E.; Wang, L. Reliability and validity of the Chinese version of the caregiver reaction assessment. *Psychiatry Clin. Neurosci.* **2011**, *65*, 254–263. [CrossRef]
25. Pallant, J. *SPSS Survival Manual: A Step by Step Guide to Data Analysis Using SPSS*; Routledge: London, UK, 2020.
26. Sperber, N.R.; Boucher, N.A.; Delgado, R.; Shepherd-Banigan, M.E.; McKenna, K.; Moore, M.; Barrett, R.; Kabat, M.; Van Houtven, C.H. Including family caregivers in seriously ill veterans' care: A mixed-methods study. *Health Aff.* **2019**, *38*, 957–963. [CrossRef]
27. Cheng, J.C.; Chang, T.T.; Wang, L.W.; Liang, S.Y.; Hsu, S.C.; Wu, S.F.; Wang, T.J.; Liu, C.Y. Development and Psychometric Evaluation of the Caregiver Caregiving Self-Efficacy Scale for Family Members with Oral Cancer. *Int. J. Nurs. Pract.* **2021**, *13*, e12957. [CrossRef]
28. Chien, W.T.; Chang, W.C.; Morrissey, J. The perceived burden among Chinese family caregivers of people with schizophrenia. *J. Clin. Nurs.* **2007**, *16*, 1151–1161. [CrossRef]
29. Yoon, S.J.; Kim, J.S.; Jung, J.G.; Kim, S.S.; Kim, S. Modifiable factors associated with caregiver burden among family caregivers of terminally ill Korean cancer patients. *Support. Care Cancer* **2014**, *22*, 1243–1250. [CrossRef]
30. Sun, Y.; Ji, M.; Leng, M.; Li, X.; Zhang, X.; Wang, Z. Comparative efficacy of 11 non-pharmacological interventions on depression, anxiety, quality of life, and caregiver burden for informal caregivers of people with dementia: A systematic review and network meta-analysis. *Int. J. Nurs. Stud.* **2022**, *129*, 104204. [CrossRef]
31. Basu, R.; Hochhalter, A.K.; Stevens, A.B. The impact of the REACH II intervention on caregivers' perceived health. *J. Appl. Gerontol.* **2015**, *34*, 590–608. [CrossRef]
32. Berwig, M.; Heinrich, S.; Spahlholz, J.; Hallensleben, N.; Brähler, E.; Gertz, H.J. Individualized support for informal caregivers of people with dementia-effectiveness of the German adaptation of REACH II. *BMC Geriatr.* **2017**, *17*, 286. [CrossRef]
33. Czaja, S.J.; Loewenstein, D.; Schulz, R.; Nair, S.N.; Perdomo, D. A videophone psychosocial intervention for dementia caregivers. *Am. J. Geriatr. Psychiatry* **2013**, *21*, 1071–1081. [CrossRef]
34. Belle, S.H.; Burgio, L.; Burns, R.; Coon, D.; Czaja, S.J.; Gallagher-Thompson, D.; Gitlin, L.N.; Klinger, J.; Koepke, K.M.; Lee, C.C.; et al. Enhancing the quality of life of dementia caregivers from different ethnic or racial groups: A randomized, controlled trial. *Ann. Intern. Med.* **2006**, *145*, 727–738. [CrossRef]
35. Cheng, S.T.; Lam, L.C.W.; Kwok, T.; Ng, N.S.S.; Fung, A.W.T. The social networks of hong kong chinese family caregivers of alzheimer's disease: Correlates with positive gains and burden. *Gerontologist* **2013**, *53*, 998–1008. [CrossRef]
36. Balard, F.; Gely-Nargeot, M.C.; Corvol, A.; Saint-Jean, O.; Somme, D. Case management for the elderly with complex needs: Cross-linking the views of their role held by elderly people, their informal caregivers and the case managers. *BMC Health Serv. Res.* **2016**, *16*, 635. [CrossRef]

Disclaimer/Publisher's Note: The statements, opinions and data contained in all publications are solely those of the individual author(s) and contributor(s) and not of MDPI and/or the editor(s). MDPI and/or the editor(s) disclaim responsibility for any injury to people or property resulting from any ideas, methods, instructions or products referred to in the content.

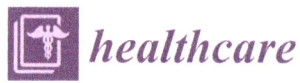

Brief Report

Caregiver Burden among Family Caregivers of Cancer Survivors Aged 75 Years or Older in Japan: A Pilot Study

Yoshiko Kitamura [1,*], Hisao Nakai [1], Yukie Maekawa [2], Hisako Yonezawa [2], Kazuko Kitamura [3], Tomoe Hashimoto [1] and Yoshiharu Motoo [3]

1 School of Nursing, Kanazawa Medical University, Kahoku 920-0293, Japan
2 Kanazawa Medical University Hospital, Kahoku 920-0293, Japan
3 Komatsu Sophia Hospital, Komatsu 923-0861, Japan
* Correspondence: kitamu@kanazawa-med.ac.jp; Tel.: +81-76-286-2211 (ext. 37568)

Abstract: The purpose of this study was to assess the burden of caregiving among family caregivers of cancer survivors aged 75 years or older in Japan. We included family caregivers of cancer survivors aged 75 years or older who were attending two hospitals in Ishikawa Prefecture, Japan, or receiving treatment during home visits. A self-administered questionnaire was developed based on previous studies. We obtained 37 responses from 37 respondents. Excluding those with incomplete responses, we had data from 35 respondents for analysis. The factor that significantly influenced the burden of caregiving for cancer survivors aged 75 years or older and family caregivers living together was the provision of full-time care ($p = 0.041$). Helping cancer survivors manage money ($p = 0.055$) was also associated with a higher burden. For family caregivers living separately, a more detailed examination of the association between the sense of caregiving burden and distance of travel to provide home-visit care is necessary, along with more support to attend hospitals with cancer survivors.

Keywords: family caregivers; caregiver burden; cancer survivors; aged; Japan

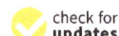

Citation: Kitamura, Y.; Nakai, H.; Maekawa, Y.; Yonezawa, H.; Kitamura, K.; Hashimoto, T.; Motoo, Y. Caregiver Burden among Family Caregivers of Cancer Survivors Aged 75 Years or Older in Japan: A Pilot Study. *Healthcare* **2023**, *11*, 473. https://doi.org/10.3390/healthcare11040473

Academic Editor: Qiuping Li

Received: 21 December 2022
Revised: 2 February 2023
Accepted: 3 February 2023
Published: 6 February 2023

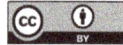

Copyright: © 2023 by the authors. Licensee MDPI, Basel, Switzerland. This article is an open access article distributed under the terms and conditions of the Creative Commons Attribution (CC BY) license (https://creativecommons.org/licenses/by/4.0/).

1. Introduction

The number of people aged 65 and over is increasing worldwide. The average life expectancy in the world has increased by more than 8 years since 1990, reaching 72.6 years in 2019 and is expected to reach 77.1 years by 2050 [1]. When older people become frail, families are often the first to provide care, and many of these family members are likely to be working [2]. Family caregivers often provide informal and unpaid care [3–6], frequently living with the care recipient, and spending a lot of time caring for them [3,4]. However, they may not be able to provide all the care needed. They may also experience both a physical and psychological burden that may affect their health. Those caring for a family member with an irreversible and progressive illness, particularly dementia, may experience a deterioration in their health, including a nervous breakdown and sleep disturbances [7,8]. Caring for a family member with Alzheimer's disease can cause stress, anxiety, and depression in family caregivers [9]. Those who care for older people with mental health problems, provide long-term care, and have little social support are at increased risk of mental health problems themselves, including depression [10,11]. A study in a Thai rural community found that the predictors of caregiver burden were the care recipient's ability to perform activities of daily living, the depression score of the caregiver, and the total hours of care provided [12]. The employment status of family caregivers has also been cited as a predictor of the care burden of older adults [13]. The burden of caregiving for working family caregivers includes both the direct burden of caregiving, and changes in their roles and employment, as well as schedule disruptions due to frequent visits to hospitals and clinics [14]. The caregiver burden is therefore affected by whether family caregivers are working.

The number of cancer survivors continues to increase because of advances in early detection and treatment and the aging and growth of the population [15]. Estimates to the year 2035 indicate that the number of older cancer survivors may increase worldwide. The largest relative increases in incidence are predicted in the Middle East and Northern Africa (+157%), and China (+155%) [16]. Older cancer survivors often have underlying medical conditions in addition to cancer and require complex healthcare provisions. This places a high demand on their caregivers [17]. The burden on family caregivers may also be affected by the increasing immobility of cancer patients if their condition deteriorates [18]. Family caregivers who spend a lot of time with cancer patients have been shown to experience psychological and physical health problems due to the strain and burden of caregiving [19]. Caregivers caring for a cancer patient while raising children, and working family caregivers may also experience their own physical and psychological health issues [20].

The aging of the population in Japan is progressing at a rate unparalleled in other countries. The proportion of people over 65 years old in Japan is 28.8% [21], and cancer is the most common cause of death among all Japanese and those over 75 years old [22]. The number of older people in Japan is expected to continue to increase until 2036 [21]. The life expectancy of cancer survivors is also improving [23]. Caring for cancer survivors is therefore a serious issue. The number of older people living alone or in married-couple households is also increasing in Japan [24], and the number of adult children living apart from their parents but still providing care is increasing.

The purpose of this study was to understand the burden of caregiving among family caregivers of cancer survivors aged 75 years or older in Japan. This study was also a pilot study for a future survey. We will determine the survey questions from this study. The survey will then aim to clarify the characteristics of family caregivers and their sense of burden in caring for cancer survivors aged 75 years or older who are living at home in Ishikawa Prefecture, Japan.

2. Materials and Methods

2.1. Study Design and Participants

This was a cross-sectional study using self-administered questionnaires. We included family caregivers of cancer survivors aged 75 years or older who were attending two hospitals that provide care for cancer survivors in Ishikawa Prefecture, Japan, or receiving treatment during home visits. Family caregivers were invited to participate by physicians from the two hospitals. Ishikawa Prefecture is in the center of the Hokuriku region facing the Sea of Japan, with the Noto peninsula jutting out into the Sea of Japan to the north [25]. The population of Ishikawa Prefecture is approximately 1.12 million, and around 30% of them are over 65 years old [26].

2.2. Data Collection

For this study, we developed a self-administered questionnaire based on previous studies. We used the Lawton Instrumental Activities of Daily Living [27] as a reference to investigate the care provided by family caregivers with activities of daily living of cancer survivors aged 75 years or older. The Burden Index of Caregiver-11 (BIC-11) was used to measure the sense of caregiving burden. The BIC-11 is a multidimensional scale that measures the sense of burden among caregivers who care for someone at home. The BIC-11 was created as a unique Japanese caregiver burden scale. The scale consists of five domains: time-dependent burden, emotional burden, existential burden, physical burden, and service-related burden. Each domain consists of two questions and 10 sub-items. This gives a total of 11 items, including the total care burden [28]. The total score ranges from 0 to 44, with higher scores indicating a greater burden on family caregivers [29]. The validity and reliability of the BIC-11 have been confirmed [28]. This study was conducted from 1 March to 31 March 2022.

2.3. Survey Details

2.3.1. Family Caregivers' Background

The basic attributes taken about family caregivers were age and sex. We also asked them whether they were living with the cancer survivor to whom they provided care using the options: "living together" or "living separately". Their options for employment type were "full-time", "part-time", "unemployed", or "other". Annual income was classified into three categories based on the distribution of the annual income of older people's households in Japan: "less than 3.18 million yen", "between 3.18 million yen and 3.48 million yen", and "3.48 million yen or more" [30]. Health status was categorized as "good", "fairly good", "somewhat poor" and "poor". Respondents were asked to indicate whether they had any chronic conditions using three options: "yes", "no" and "don't know".

2.3.2. Background of Cancer Survivors Aged 75 Years and Older

The caregivers were asked to provide information about the basic attributes of their care recipient, such as their age, sex, and relationship with the family caregiver. Respondents selected treatment history by treatment method from "surgery", "radiation therapy", "chemotherapy", and "other". They were also asked whether the care recipient had any diseases other than cancer using, responding "yes", "no", or "don't know". We also asked if the care recipient had a diagnosis of dementia (possible responses were "yes", "no", and "don't know").

2.3.3. Family Caregiver Care Status

The respondents were asked how long they had been taking care of family members; there were four response categories: "less than 1 year", "1–3 years", "3–5 years", and "5 years or more". Respondents were asked about the number of times they had to get up at night to provide care in the past month; there were four categories: "often", "sometimes", "almost never", and "never". The respondents were asked if they had experienced difficulties doing other household chores and jobs because of caregiving in the past month; there were four categories: "often", "sometimes", "almost never", and "never". Respondents were asked about care partners and care advisors, both with responses of "present" or "absent".

2.3.4. Family Caregiver Care Details

The respondents were asked to answer "yes" or "no" to say if they provided help with "making phone calls", "shopping", "meal preparation", "eating meals", "cleaning", "dressing", "bathing", "using the toilet", "defecation (including handling enemas and suppositories)", "urination (including handling the urinal)", "changing clothes", "laundry", "transportation to and from to hospital", "walking (including accompanying and operating wheelchair)", "getting in or out of bed", "medication management", "money management", and "advising about concerns".

2.3.5. Family Caregivers' Sense of Caregiving Burden

The BIC-11 was used to assess family caregivers' sense of caregiving burden. Items included: "I don't have enough time for myself because of caregiving", "I can't go out freely because of caregiving", "I get tired of everything when I am a caregiver", "I want to leave caregiving to someone else", "It is hard because I don't feel fulfilled when I am a caregiver", "It is hard because I don't find meaning in caring for my family member", "I feel physical pain when providing care", "My health has suffered because of caregiving", "I don't feel like caring for my family member", and "I feel like I want to leave the work to someone else". Other items include "I am troubled because patients do not want caregiving services", "It is a burden that caregiving services come into my house" and "Overall, how much of a burden do you think caregiving is on you?". All responses used a five-point Likert-type scale (0 = never, 1 = almost never, 2 = sometimes, 3 = often, 4 = always).

2.3.6. Support Required by Family Caregivers

The respondents were asked to comment freely on the support they required.

2.4. Analysis Methods

After obtaining the distribution of the background of family caregivers and cancer survivors aged 75 years or older, we defined the employment type of family caregivers as "full-time" for those who answered "full-time" and "other" for all other responses. Annual income was defined as "less than 3.18 million yen" for "less than 3.18 million yen" and "other" for all other responses. Health status was classified into two categories: general health status into "good" for "good/fairly good" and "other" for "somewhat poor/poor", and chronic conditions into "yes" for those who responded "yes", and "other" for responses of "no" or "don't know". The background of cancer survivors aged 75 years or older were analyzed by classifying a diagnosis of dementia into "yes" and "other" (for responses of "no/don't know"). The duration of care was "less than 1 year" and "other" (for "1–3 years", "3–5 years", and "5 years or more"). Respondents who answered "often/sometimes" to the number of times they had to get up at night to provide care in the past month were grouped into "yes", and those who answered "almost never/never" into "other". BIC-11 uses a five-point Likert-type scale (0 = never, 1 = almost never, 2 = sometimes, 3 = often, 4 = always). After obtaining the distribution of the BIC-11 scores, we divided the group into two using the median value, giving a no or low care burden group and a high care burden group, in line with a previous study [31].

Overall, 32 (91.4%) of the study participants lived with a cancer survivor aged 75 years or older. Three family caregivers (8.6%) who lived separately were excluded to control for the effect of residential status on the burden of caregiving. We used the chi-square test or Fisher's direct probability test to examine the association between the other items and the sense of caregiving burden of family caregivers living with the care recipient as an objective variable. The significance level was set at 5%. We used SPSS Ver. 27 (IBM Corp., Armonk, NY, USA) for statistical analysis. The support currently required by family caregivers was categorized by the type of residence.

2.5. Ethical Considerations

This study was carried out with the approval of the University Medical Research Ethics Review Committees at the authors' universities (No. I692). The participants were given a written informed consent form and were informed of the purpose and importance of the study, the survey method, the fact that participation was voluntary, and the fact that they would not be personally identified when the results were made public. Participants completed a self-administered questionnaire. Completion of the questionnaire implied their consent.

3. Results

Overall, 60 family caregivers were asked to participate in the survey and 37 responded (response rate: 61.7%), with 35 respondents (94.6%) answering all the items. The mean age (standard deviation) of the family caregivers was 68.9 (11.1) years, four were men (11.4%), and 31 were women (88.6%). For living arrangements, 32 (91.4%) were living with their care recipient and three (8.6%) separately. The mean (standard deviation) age of cancer survivors over 75 years was 79.9 (4.1) years, 27 (77.1%) were men and eight (22.9%) were women. The backgrounds of family caregivers and cancer survivors are shown in Table 1.

Table 1. Background of family caregivers and cancer survivors over 75 years (n = 35).

Item		n	(%)
Family caregiver background			
Age (median [range]), years	74.0 (47–82)		
Sex	Men	4	(11.4)
	Women	31	(88.6)
Living arrangements with cancer survivors aged 75 years and older	Living together	32	(91.4)
	Living separately	3	(8.6)
Background of cancer survivors aged 75 years and older			
Age (median [range]), years	79.0 (75–95)		
Sex	Men	27	(77.1)
	Women	8	(22.9)
Relationship with family caregiver			
	Husband	23	(65.7)
	Mother	8	(22.9)
	Father	3	(8.6)
	Father-in-law	1	(2.9)
Treatment history by treatment method (multiple answers allowed)			
	Chemotherapy	27	(77.1)
	Surgery	16	(45.7)
	Radiation therapy	11	(31.4)
	Other	1	(2.9)
Diseases other than cancer	Yes	13	(37.1)
	Other	22	(62.9)

3.1. Factors Associated with BIC-11 Score of Family Caregivers Living with the Care Recipient (n = 32)

Overall, 32 family caregivers were living with the cancer survivor, and their mean age (standard deviation) was 70.4 (10.0) years. They included three men (8.4%) and 29 women (90.6%). The median (range) of BIC-11 was 2.0 (0–28). The distribution of BIC-11 was 0 = 12 (37.5%), 1 = 3 (9.4%), 2 = 3 (9.4%), and ≥ 3 = 14 (43.7%). The results of the univariate analysis are shown in Table 2. Eight (25.0%) full-time employees (p = 0.041) had a significantly higher percentage of high BIC-11, as did the 12 respondents (37.5%) who provided money management help for cancer survivors (p = 0.055). Table 2 shows the results of the cross-tabulation.

3.2. Background of Family Caregivers Living Separately from the Care Recipient (n = 3)

The mean age (standard deviation) was 50.7 years (3.2). There was one man (33.3%) and two women (66.7%).

3.3. Support Required by Family Caregivers (Free Answer) (n = 3)

The family caregivers who lived with their fathers indicated that they needed information about available caregiver support as soon as possible, to be listened to, and to have support with helping the caregiver to take baths and for housework. The family caregivers who lived apart from their cancer survivors mentioned that they needed help to reduce the burden of taking their care recipient to and from the doctor's office once a week, which took 3 h each way, transportation expenses for visiting the doctor, and support for accompanying the care recipients when they visit the doctor.

Table 2. Background and caregiving status of family caregivers and cancer survivors in relation to BIC-11 (n = 32).

Item	Category	Total n	(%)	Burden of Care (BIC-11) No or Low Group n	(%)	High Group n	(%)	p Value
Family caregiver's basic attributes, work status, annual income, health status, pre-existing conditions								
Age	Average	32	(100.0)	15	(46.9)	17	(53.1)	0.389 [1]
Sex	Men	3	(9.4)	1	(33.3)	2	(66.7)	1.000 [2]
	Women	29	(90.6)	14	(48.3)	15	(51.7)	
Employment type	Full-time	8	(25.0)	1	(12.5)	7	(87.5)	0.041 [2]
	Other	24	(75.0)	14	(58.3)	10	(41.7)	
Annual income	Less than 3.18 million yen	24	(75.0)	13	(54.2)	11	(45.8)	0.229 [2]
	Other	8	(25.0)	2	(25.0)	6	(75.0)	
Status of health	Good	24	(75.0)	11	(45.8)	13	(54.2)	1.000 [2]
	Other	8	(25.0)	4	(50.0)	4	(50.0)	
Chronic conditions	Yes	12	(37.5)	6	(50.0)	6	(50.0)	0.784 [1]
	Other	20	(62.5)	9	(45.0)	11	(55.0)	
Attributes of cancer survivors aged 75 years or older								
Age	Average	32	(100.0)	15	(46.9)	17	(53.1)	0.433 [1]
Sex	Men	25	(78.1)	11	(44.0)	14	(56.0)	0.424 [2]
	Women	7	(21.9)	4	(57.1)	3	(42.9)	
Diagnosis of dementia	Yes	3	(9.4)	1	(33.3)	2	(66.7)	1.000 [2]
	Other	29	(90.6)	14	(48.3)	15	(51.7)	
Family caregiver status								
Period providing care	Less than 1 year	16	(50.0)	8	(50.0)	8	(50.0)	0.723 [1]
	Other	16	(50.0)	7	(43.8)	9	(56.3)	
In the past month, have you had to get up at night to provide care?	Yes	6	(18.8)	1	(16.7)	5	(83.3)	0.178 [2]
	Other	26	(81.3)	14	(53.8)	12	(46.2)	
In the past month, has caregiving made it difficult for you to do other household chores or jobs?	Yes	9	(28.1)	6	(66.7)	3	(33.3)	0.243 [2]
	Other	23	(71.9)	9	(39.1)	14	(60.9)	

Table 2. Cont.

Item	Category	Total n	(%)	Burden of Care (BIC-11)				p Value
				No or Low Group n	(%)	High Group n	(%)	
Care partners	Present	24	(75.0)	12	(50.0)	12	(50.0)	0.691 [2]
	Absent	8	(25.0)	3	(37.5)	5	(62.5)	
Care advisors	Present	27	(84.4)	14	(51.9)	13	(48.1)	0.338 [2]
	Absent	5	(15.6)	1	(20.0)	4	(80.0)	
Care provided by family caregiver								
Making phone calls	Yes	9	(28.1)	3	(33.3)	6	(66.7)	0.444 [2]
	No	23	(71.9)	12	(52.2)	11	(47.8)	
Shopping	Yes	10	(31.3)	5	(50.0)	5	(50.0)	1.000 [2]
	No	22	(68.8)	10	(45.5)	12	(54.5)	
Meal preparation	Yes	22	(68.8)	9	(40.9)	13	(59.1)	0.450 [2]
	No	10	(31.3)	6	(60.0)	4	(40.0)	
Eating meals	Yes	4	(12.5)	2	(50.0)	2	(50.0)	1.000 [2]
	No	28	(87.5)	13	(46.4)	15	(53.6)	
Cleaning	Yes	16	(50.0)	6	(37.5)	10	(62.5)	0.288 [1]
	No	16	(50.0)	9	(56.3)	7	(43.8)	
Dressing	Yes	3	(9.4)	1	(33.3)	2	(66.7)	1.000 [2]
	No	29	(90.6)	14	(48.3)	15	(51.7)	
Bathing	Yes	5	(15.6)	4	(80.0)	1	(20.0)	0.161 [2]
	No	27	(84.4)	11	(40.7)	16	(59.3)	
Using the toilet	Yes	5	(15.6)	2	(40.0)	3	(60.0)	1.000 [2]
	No	27	(84.4)	13	(48.1)	14	(51.9)	
Defecation (including handling enemas and suppositories)	Yes	2	(6.3)	1	(50.0)	1	(50.0)	1.000 [2]
	No	30	(93.8)	14	(46.7)	16	(53.3)	
Urination (including handling the urinal)	Yes	3	(9.4)	1	(33.3)	2	(66.7)	1.000 [2]
	No	29	(90.6)	14	(48.3)	15	(51.7)	

Table 2. Cont.

Item	Category	Total		Burden of Care (BIC-11)				p Value
				No or Low Group		High Group		
		n	(%)	n	(%)	n	(%)	
Changing clothes	Yes	7	(21.9)	3	(42.9)	4	(57.1)	1.000 [2]
	No	25	(78.1)	12	(48.0)	13	(52.0)	
Laundry	Yes	19	(59.4)	9	(47.4)	10	(52.6)	0.946 [1]
	No	13	(40.6)	6	(46.2)	7	(53.8)	
Transportation to and from the hospital	Yes	12	(37.5)	6	(50.0)	6	(50.0)	0.784 [1]
	No	20	(62.5)	9	(45.0)	11	(55.0)	
Walking (including accompanying and operating wheelchair)	Yes	2	(6.3)	2	(100.0)	0	(0.0)	0.212 [2]
	No	30	(93.8)	13	(43.3)	17	(56.7)	
Getting in or out of bed	Yes	3	(9.4)	1	(33.3)	2	(66.7)	1.000 [2]
	No	29	(90.6)	14	(48.3)	15	(51.7)	
Medication management	Yes	12	(37.5)	5	(41.7)	7	(58.3)	0.647 [1]
	No	20	(62.5)	10	(50.0)	10	(50.0)	
Money management	Yes	12	(37.5)	3	(25.0)	9	(75.0)	0.055 [1]
	No	20	(62.5)	12	(60.0)	8	(40.0)	
Advising about concerns	Yes	7	(21.9)	3	(42.9)	4	(57.1)	1.000 [2]
	No	25	(78.1)	12	(48.0)	13	(52.0)	

[1] χ^2 test, [2] Fisher's exact test.

4. Discussion

Our study aimed to understand the burden of caregiving among family caregivers of cancer survivors aged 75 years or older who receive home care, hospital visits, or home visits in Ishikawa Prefecture, Japan. The mean age of the participants in the study by Sugiyama et al. on family caregivers with Japanese cancer survivors was 48 years [32]. The mean age of the participants in this study was 68.9 years, which may have been influenced by the fact that this study was conducted among family caregivers of cancer survivors aged 75 years or more.

Many studies have reported the relationship between employment and family caregivers' sense of caregiving burden [33–36]. In particular, it has been pointed out that the physical functions of cancer patients decline at the end of life, which makes family caregivers more anxious, increases their sense of caregiving burden, and has a negative effect on their employment [37,38]. In our study, working full-time was associated with a high care burden, but the direction of the relationship is unclear. However, full-time work may be an important factor when considering the burden of providing care.

When older adults rely on their children for financial support and caregiving, their children's physical and mental health is threatened and family relationships are negatively affected [39,40]. We found that providing money management support was associated with an increased burden among family caregivers. It is not clear why this should be the case, and this will need further investigation in future studies.

One free text comment from family caregivers who lived apart from their care recipient noted that the 3-h each-way trip by private car and long outpatient visits were a burden. In a previous study, the average distance traveled by cancer survivors aged 75 years or older to receive outpatient chemotherapy in Ishikawa Prefecture, Japan, was 40.7 km [41]. In Japan, the physical burden and fatigue of patients who travel long distances to receive outpatient chemotherapy are issues [42]. Our findings suggest that long-distance travel may also be a burden for family caregivers who live separately. Only three family caregivers were living apart from their cancer survivors, so the relationship with caregiver burden is unknown at this time, but those who support cancer survivors need to be aware of the burden on caregivers of providing care and attending long outpatient visits with the patient.

Previous results suggest that family caregivers are also older and at risk of developing cancer themselves [43]. Another study found that the improved life expectancy of cancer survivors [23] means it is necessary to clarify the burden of family caregivers who work full-time, manage the money of the cancer survivor, and travel to the cancer survivor's home from neighboring cities to provide care. Our study supports these findings.

This study had several limitations. First, the total number of respondents was small. Only three family caregivers lived separately from their care recipients. Second, most of the results have a gender bias, because the majority of caregivers were female (88.6%). Third, the majority of study participants were family caregivers living with their cancer survivors and with a low caregiving burden. Many of the cancer survivors over 75 years of age living with their caregivers may have had a good ability to perform activities of daily living and therefore presented a low physical caregiving burden. Fourth, the BIC-11 is a scale suitable for measuring the burden of caregivers who care for a family member at home [28]. It may not be suitable for measuring the burden of caregiving among family caregivers of cancer survivors. Fifth, information on cancer survivors was reported by the family caregivers, and not the cancer survivors themselves, which may have introduced some bias or inaccuracy. Sixth, this was a cross-sectional study, and it is therefore not possible to establish any causal relationships between the study variables.

5. Conclusions

Our findings indicate that working full-time and helping cancer survivors with money management may be associated with a care burden. The distance traveled by family caregivers to provide care may also be a factor. In the future, it will be necessary to investigate the sense of caregiving burden by considering patterns of work and money management support for cancer survivors among family caregivers who live with their cancer survivors. Additionally, the number of participants should be increased to include younger caregivers and urban and rural caregivers. The method of measuring the sense of caregiving burden also needs to be re-examined. The number of older cancer survivors living alone or in married-couple households is increasing in Japan. The relationship between the distance traveled by family caregivers to provide care and support, especially with hospital visits, and their sense of caregiver burden should therefore be investigated.

Author Contributions: Conceptualization, Y.K., H.N., Y.M. (Yukie Maekawa), H.Y., T.H. and Y.M. (Yoshiharu Motoo); methodology, Y.K. and H.N.; software, Y.K.; formal analysis, Y.K. and H.N.; investigation, Y.K., Y.M. (Yukie Maekawa), H.Y., K.K. and T.H.; data curation, Y.K.; writing–original draft preparation, Y.K. and H.N.; writing–review and editing, Y.K. and H.N.; supervision, H.N.; project administration, Y.K.; funding acquisition, Y.K. All authors have read and agreed to the published version of the manuscript.

Funding: This research was supported by the 35th Research Grant (2021), Hokkoku Cancer Foundation, and KAKENHI JSP grant number [18K17537].

Institutional Review Board Statement: This research was conducted in accordance with the Declaration of Helsinki, 1995 (as revised in Seoul, 2008) and carried out with the consent of the university medical research ethics review committees at the authors' universities (No. I692).

Informed Consent Statement: Informed consent was obtained from all participants in this study.

Data Availability Statement: The data analyzed during this study are included in this published article. Further inquiries can be directed to the corresponding authors.

Acknowledgments: We thank the participants, the doctors of Kanazawa Medical University Hospital, and the doctors and nurses of Komatsu Sophia Hospital for their cooperation. We also thank Melissa Leffler for editing a draft of this manuscript.

Conflicts of Interest: The authors declare no conflict of interest.

References

1. United Nations World Population Prospects 2019: Highlights. Available online: https://population.un.org/wpp/Publications/Files/wpp2019_10KeyFindings.pdf (accessed on 6 December 2022).
2. Jin, K.; Simpkins, J.W.; Ji, X.; Leis, M.; Stambler, I. The Critical Need to Promote Research of Aging and Aging-Related Diseases to Improve Health and Longevity of the Elderly Population. *Aging Dis.* **2014**, *6*, 1–5. [CrossRef]
3. Adelman, R.D.; Tmanova, L.L.; Delgado, D.; Dion, S.; Lachs, M.S. Caregiver Burden: A Clinical Review. *JAMA* **2014**, *311*, 1052–1060. [CrossRef]
4. Li, Q.; Loke, A.Y. A Spectrum of Hidden Morbidities among Spousal Caregivers for Patients with Cancer, and Differences between the Genders: A Review of the Literature. *Eur. J. Oncol. Nurs.* **2013**, *17*, 578–587. [CrossRef]
5. Del Molero Jurado, M.M.; Pérez-Fuentes, M.D.C.; Barragán Martín, A.B.; Soriano Sánchez, J.G.; Oropesa Ruiz, N.F.; Sisto, M.; Gázquez Linares, J.J. Mindfulness in Family Caregivers of Persons with Dementia: Systematic Review and Meta-Analysis. *Healthcare* **2020**, *8*, 193. [CrossRef] [PubMed]
6. Capistrant, B.D. Caregiving for Older Adults and the Caregivers' Health: An Epidemiologic Review. *Curr. Epidemiol. Rep.* **2016**, *3*, 72–80. [CrossRef]
7. Ryan, A.A.; Scullion, H.F. Nursing Home Placement: An Exploration of the Experiences of Family Carers. *J. Adv. Nurs.* **2000**, *32*, 1187–1195. [CrossRef] [PubMed]
8. Graneheim, U.H.; Johansson, A.; Lindgren, B.-M. Family Caregivers' Experiences of Relinquishing the Care of a Person with Dementia to a Nursing Home: Insights from a Meta-Ethnographic Study. *Scand. J. Caring Sci.* **2014**, *28*, 215–224. [CrossRef]
9. Manzini, C.S.S.; Vale, F.A.C.D. Emotional Disorders Evidenced by Family Caregivers of Older People with Alzheimer's Disease. *Dement. Neuropsychol.* **2020**, *14*, 56–61. [CrossRef]
10. Baillie, V.; Norbeck, J.S.; Barnes, A.L.E. Stress, Social Support, and Psychological Distress of Family Caregivers of the Elderly. *Nurs. Res.* **1988**, *37*, 217–222. [CrossRef]
11. Chan, S.W. Global Perspective of Burden of Family Caregivers for Persons with Schizophrenia. *Arch. Psychiatr. Nurs.* **2011**, *25*, 339–349. [CrossRef]
12. Tuttle, D.; Griffiths, J.; Kaunnil, A. Predictors of Caregiver Burden in Caregivers of Older People with Physical Disabilities in a Rural Community. *PLoS ONE* **2022**, *17*, e0277177. [CrossRef]
13. So, M.K.P.; Yuk, H.; Tiwari, A.; Cheung, S.T.Y.; Chu, A.M.Y. Predicting the Burden of Family Caregivers from Their Individual Characteristics. *Inform. Health Soc. Care* **2022**, *47*, 211–222. [CrossRef]

14. Haley, W. Family Caregivers of Elderly Patients with Cancer: Understanding and Minimizing the Burden of Care. *J. Support. Oncol.* **2002**, *1*, 25–29.
15. Miller, K.D.; Siegel, R.L.; Lin, C.C.; Mariotto, A.B.; Kramer, J.L.; Rowland, J.H.; Stein, K.D.; Alteri, R.; Jemal, A. Cancer Treatment and Survivorship Statistics, 2016. *CA. Cancer J. Clin.* **2016**, *66*, 271–289. [CrossRef]
16. Pilleron, S.; Sarfati, D.; Janssen-Heijnen, M.; Vignat, J.; Ferlay, J.; Bray, F.; Soerjomataram, I. Global Cancer Incidence in Older Adults, 2012 and 2035: A Population-Based Study. *Int. J. Cancer* **2019**, *144*, 49–58. [CrossRef]
17. Etters, L.; Goodall, D.; Harrison, B.E. Caregiver Burden among Dementia Patient Caregivers: A Review of the Literature. *J. Am. Acad. Nurse Pract.* **2008**, *20*, 423–428. [CrossRef]
18. Kurtz, M.E.; Given, C.W.; Given, B.A.; Kurtz, J.C. The Interaction of Age, Symptoms, and Survival Status on Physical and Mental Health of Patients with Cancer and Their Families. *Cancer* **1994**, *74*, 2071–2078. [CrossRef]
19. Honea, N.J. Putting Evidence into Practice®: Nursing Assessment and Interventions to Reduce Family Caregiver Strain and Burden. *Clin. J. Oncol. Nurs.* **2008**, *12*, 507–516. [CrossRef]
20. Rowland, J.H.; Bellizzi, K.M. Cancer Survivorship Issues: Life After Treatment and Implications for an Aging Population. *J. Clin. Oncol.* **2014**, *32*, 2662–2668. [CrossRef]
21. Cabinet Office. Annual Report on the Ageing Society [Summary] FY2021. Available online: https://www8.cao.go.jp/kourei/english/annualreport/2021/pdf/2021.pdf (accessed on 7 December 2022).
22. Ministry of Health, Labour and Welfare Policy Report (about Cancer Control). Available online: https://www.mhlw.go.jp/seisaku/24.html (accessed on 6 December 2022). (In Japanese)
23. Brenner, H. Long-Term Survival Rates of Cancer Patients Achieved by the End of the 20th Century: A Period Analysis. *Lancet* **2002**, *360*, 1131–1135. [CrossRef]
24. Statistics Bureau of Japan 2000 Census, 8. Older Single-Person Households, 9. Older Couple Household. Available online: https://www.stat.go.jp/data/kokusei/2000/kihon1/00/09.html (accessed on 6 December 2022). (In Japanese)
25. Ishikawa Prefecture Ishikawa Prefecture Overview of Ishikawa Prefecture. Available online: http://www.pref.ishikawa.lg.jp/sabou/1gaiyou/index.html (accessed on 8 December 2022). (In Japanese)
26. Ishikawa Prefecture Ishikawa Prefecture Part 2 Current Status and Estimates of Older People Who Need Long-Term Care. 2018. (In Japanese)
27. Graf, C. The Lawton Instrumental Activities of Daily Living (IADL) Scale. Available online: https://www.alz.org/careplanning/downloads/lawton-iadl.pdf (accessed on 7 December 2022).
28. Miyashita, M.; Yamaguchi, A.; Kayama, M.; Narita, Y.; Kawada, N.; Akiyama, M.; Hagiwara, A.; Suzukamo, Y.; Fukuhara, S. Validation of the Burden Index of Caregivers (BIC), a Multidimensional Short Care Burden Scale from Japan. *Health Qual. Life Outcomes* **2006**, *4*, 52. [CrossRef] [PubMed]
29. Hanemoto, T.; Hikichi, Y.; Kikuchi, N.; Kozawa, T. The Impact of Different Anti-Vascular Endothelial Growth Factor Treatment Regimens on Reducing Burden for Caregivers and Patients with Wet Age-Related Macular Degeneration in a Single-Center Real-World Japanese Setting. *PLoS ONE* **2017**, *12*, e0189035. Available online: https://journals.plos.org/plosone/article?id=10.1371/journal.pone.0189035 (accessed on 6 December 2022). [CrossRef] [PubMed]
30. Ministry of Health, Labour and Welfare Overview of the 1997 Basic Survey of Living Conditions, 6. The Average Income of Elderly Households Is 3.16 Million Yen, of Which 62.5% Are Public Pensions. Available online: https://www.mhlw.go.jp/www1/toukei/ks-tyosa/1-2-6.html (accessed on 6 December 2022). (In Japanese)
31. Changes in the Quality of Life of Patients with Left Ventricular Assist Device and Their Caregivers in Japan: Retrospective Observational Study. Available online: https://www.jstage.jst.go.jp/article/tjem/257/1/257_2022.J016/_article (accessed on 6 December 2022).
32. Sugiyama, I.; Shoji, H.; Igarashi, N.; Sato, K.; Takahashi, M.; Miyashita, M. Factors Affecting Quality of Life of Family Caregivers of Cancer Patients: Study Using the Japanese Version CQOLC (The Caregiver Quality of Life Index-Cancer). *Palliat. Care Res.* **2017**, *12*, 259–269. (In Japanese) [CrossRef]
33. Otis-Green, S.; Juarez, G. Enhancing the Social Well-Being of Family Caregivers. *Semin. Oncol. Nurs.* **2012**, *28*, 246–255. [CrossRef]
34. Kim, Y.; Given, B.A. Quality of Life of Family Caregivers of Cancer Survivors. *Cancer* **2008**, *112*, 2556–2568. [CrossRef]
35. Blum, K.; Sherman, D.W. Understanding the Experience of Caregivers: A Focus on Transitions. *Semin. Oncol. Nurs.* **2010**, *26*, 243–258. [CrossRef]
36. Given, B.A.; Given, C.W.; Sherwood, P. The Challenge of Quality Cancer Care for Family Caregivers. *Semin. Oncol. Nurs.* **2012**, *28*, 205–212. [CrossRef]
37. Grunfeld, E.; Coyle, D.; Whelan, T.; Clinch, J.; Reyno, L.; Earle, C.C.; Willan, A.; Viola, R.; Coristine, M.; Janz, T.; et al. Family Caregiver Burden: Results of a Longitudinal Study of Breast Cancer Patients and Their Principal Caregivers. *CMAJ Can. Med. Assoc. J. J. Assoc. Medicale Can.* **2004**, *170*, 1795–1801. [CrossRef]
38. Palma, E.; Simonetti, V.; Franchelli, P.; Pavone, D.; Cicolini, G. An Observational Study of Family Caregivers' Quality of Life Caring for Patients with a Stoma. *Gastroenterol. Nurs.* **2012**, *35*, 99–104. [CrossRef]
39. Fisher, K.R.; Shang, X.; Li, Z. Absent Role of the State: Analysis of Social Support to Older People with Disabilities in Rural China. *Soc. Policy Adm.* **2011**, *45*, 633–648. [CrossRef]
40. Jeong, A.; Shin, D.; Park, J.H.; Park, K. Attributes of Caregivers' Quality of Life: A Perspective Comparison between Spousal and Non-Spousal Caregivers of Older Patients with Cancer. *J. Geriatr. Oncol.* **2020**, *11*, 82–87. [CrossRef]

41. Kitamura, Y.; Nakai, H.; Hashimoto, T.; Morikawa, Y.; Motoo, Y. Correlation between Quality of Life under Treatment and Current Life Satisfaction among Cancer Survivors Aged 75 Years and Older Receiving Outpatient Chemotherapy in Ishikawa Prefecture, Japan. *Healthcare* **2022**, *10*, 1863. [CrossRef]
42. Shizuoka Cancer Center Concerns of Outpatient Cancer Patients. Q&A. Available online: https://www.scchr.jp/cancerqa/jyogen_3800003.html (accessed on 6 December 2022). (In Japanese)
43. Smith, B.D.; Smith, G.L.; Hurria, A.; Hortobagyi, G.N.; Buchholz, T.A. Future of Cancer Incidence in the United States: Burdens Upon an Aging, Changing Nation. *J. Clin. Oncol.* **2009**, *27*, 2758–2765. [CrossRef]

Disclaimer/Publisher's Note: The statements, opinions and data contained in all publications are solely those of the individual author(s) and contributor(s) and not of MDPI and/or the editor(s). MDPI and/or the editor(s) disclaim responsibility for any injury to people or property resulting from any ideas, methods, instructions or products referred to in the content.

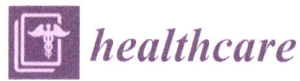

Article

Therapeutic Communication Experiences of Nurses Caring for Patients with Hematology

Hyun-Jung Lee [1], Bom-Mi Park [2,*], Mi-Jin Shin [1] and Do-Yeon Kim [1]

1. Department of Nursing, The Catholic University of Korea, Seoul ST. Mary's Hospital, Seoul 06591, Republic of Korea
2. Department of Nursing, Konkuk University, Chungju-si 27478, Republic of Korea
* Correspondence: spring0317@kku.ac.kr

Abstract: Nurses who take care of patients with hematology have more difficulty in therapeutic communication. The aim of this study is to explore the therapeutic communication experiences of nurses caring for patients with hematology and the meaning of the essential structure of therapeutic communication. Colaizzi's phenomenological method was applied to explore the essential structures and meanings of therapeutic communication in depth through a focus group interview. The interview was conducted at a tertiary care hospital with 20 nurses caring for patients with hematology. As a result of the analyses, 22 themes, 14 theme clusters, and 5 categories were derived. The categories derived from the analyses included "acquiring core competencies as nursing professionals", "improving patient-centered nursing performance", "forming a partnership treatment relationship", "obtaining clinical performance skills to solve problems", and "preparing efficient system improvement". Based on this study's results, it will be possible to provide high-quality nursing to patients by improving the therapeutic communication ability of nurses caring for patients with hematology. In addition, it will be the basis for the development of a nurses' therapeutic communication promotion program for nurses caring for such patients.

Keywords: therapeutic communication; patients with hematology; nurse; phenomenology; focus group interview

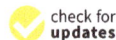

Citation: Lee, H.-J.; Park, B.-M.; Shin, M.-J.; Kim, D.-Y. Therapeutic Communication Experiences of Nurses Caring for Patients with Hematology. *Healthcare* 2022, 10, 2403. https://doi.org/10.3390/healthcare10122403

Academic Editor: Susan Letvak

Received: 18 September 2022
Accepted: 28 November 2022
Published: 30 November 2022

Publisher's Note: MDPI stays neutral with regard to jurisdictional claims in published maps and institutional affiliations.

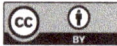

Copyright: © 2022 by the authors. Licensee MDPI, Basel, Switzerland. This article is an open access article distributed under the terms and conditions of the Creative Commons Attribution (CC BY) license (https://creativecommons.org/licenses/by/4.0/).

1. Introduction

Therapeutic communication is defined as an interaction aimed at improving the emotional and physical problems of patients [1,2]. Therapeutic communication includes open-ended questions, listening, reflection, silence, clarity, nonverbal or verbal signals, identifying and providing evidence, and summarizing the tone of emotion [3]. For nurses, in particular, communication can be considered an essential component of nursing expertise that can enable them to understand, evaluate, and focus on each patient [4,5]. A nurse's effective therapeutic communication represents their ability to know what to say and do during interactions with a patient [6]. The patients' satisfaction with hospital life varies according to the nurses' level of communication [7]. Communication increases patients' knowledge, enabling them to use self-health techniques that ultimately affect their health and well-being [8]. Ultimately, therapeutic communication between nurses and patients can foster positive treatment results through certain interactions [4].

Patients come to the hospital due to illness and suffer mentally and physically due to changes in the unfamiliar environment of the hospital [9]. Patients with hematology must accept the consequences of a life-threatening disease after the initial diagnosis as well as endure the side effects of various tests and treatments, along with changes in their living conditions and lifestyles [10]. Such patients, in particular, initially exhibit poor communication, such as avoiding talking about their disease [10]. However, the rate of progression of hematological diseases is fast, often having fatal consequences; therefore, after receiving treatment, patients may continue to rely on nurses and continuously ask questions or have concerns about the uncertain number of treatments [11]. This is because patients feel comfortable when nurses approach and talk to them, and they hope that the nurse will spend considerable time communicating with them [10]. However, in a clinical setting, patients may perceive a lack of therapeutic communication with the nurses due to the insufficient number of nurses, overwork of nurses, lack of knowledge of therapeutic communication with nurses, and the patient's own anxiety and suffering [2].

Notably, one study reported that the lack of therapeutic communication by nurses was associated with a lack of repeated acquisition of therapeutic communication skills [4]. In addition, nurses providing care to patients with hematology have difficulty communicating with patients during crisis situations, such as at the first diagnosis or if the disease recurs [12]. Moreover, during the coronavirus disease 2019 (COVID-19) pandemic, a study reported that patients perceived more barriers to communication due to the wearing of face masks [13]. Communication between patient and nurse in clinical situations occurs through interaction and may vary depending on the situation and personal characteristics [14]. Therefore, nurses should be able to communicate with patients and understand their needs and emotions [15].

Most of the advanced qualitative studies on nurses' therapeutic communication to date have focused on nurses caring for cancer patients, nursing students, and therapeutic communication by hematology oncologists; however, qualitative studies on nurses caring for hospitalized patients with hematological cancer at tertiary hospitals are scarce. Therefore, in this study, we aim to explore the essential structures and meanings of the therapeutic communication experiences of the nurses caring for patients with hematology. To elucidate the comprehensive experiences of nurses caring for patients with hematology, focus group [16] interviews, aimed at extensively exploring individual experiences, sharing ideas, and gathering opinions on common problems, were conducted, confirming nurses' difficulty in providing therapeutic communication.

2. Materials and Methods

2.1. Design

In this study, we employed focus group interviews to explore the therapeutic communication experiences of nurses experienced in caring for patients with hematological cancer. A qualitative design was adopted by applying the phenomenological method of Colaizzi [17], a rigorous and qualitative approach to finding, understanding, explaining, describing, and revealing new topics and intertwined relationships [17], to examine the structure and meaning of therapeutic communication.

2.2. Selection of Participants

Participants in this study were 20 nurses working at a tertiary care hospital in a metropolitan city in Korea who had experience caring for patients with hematological cancer. They felt keenly about communication problems with blood cancer patients and wanted to actively participate. We selected 10 nurses with more than five years of clinical experience and 10 with less than five years of clinical experience through an announcement by the Ministry of Nursing; those who fully understood this study and agreed to participate were sampled. The participants' general characteristics included age, gender, education, clinical experience with patients of a hematology cancer ward, and total clinical experience. The nurses in the ward were usually young (the median age was 29 years), and all 20 nurses were women. The nurses' educational background was a bachelor's degree or higher, and the average length of clinical experience in the hematology cancer ward was four years and eight months. Their average length of clinical experience was five years and eight months (Table 1).

Table 1. Demographic and clinical characteristics of the nurses (N = 20).

ID	Age (Year)	Gender	Education Level	Clinical Experience with Patients of Hematology-Oncology Ward (y)	Total Clinical Experience (y)
1	26	Women	Bachelor's	2.11	2.11
2	32	Women	Master's	7.11	7.11
3	31	Women	Master's	8.11	8.11
4	29	Women	Bachelor's	6.60	6.60
5	29	Women	Bachelor's	5.20	5.20
6	36	Women	Bachelor's	11.00	14.30
7	36	Women	Bachelor's	5.20	6.20
8	37	Women	Bachelor's	9.00	14.00
9	30	Women	Associate's	6.10	8.30
10	25	Women	Bachelor's	3.00	3.00
11	26	Women	Bachelor's	2.60	2.60
12	25	Women	Bachelor's	2.80	2.80
13	26	Women	Bachelor's	2.90	2.90
14	26	Women	Bachelor's	2.11	2.11
15	25	Women	Bachelor's	2.60	2.60
16	37	Women	Bachelor's	14.11	14.11
17	27	Women	Bachelor's	2.11	2.11
18	24	Women	Bachelor's	2.00	2.00
19	24	Women	Bachelor's	1.10	1.10
20	29	Women	Bachelor's	5.40	5.40

2.3. Procedure

Data collection for this study was conducted after obtaining approval from the Institutional Review Board. The researcher submitted a letter of cooperation to the tertiary care hospital's nursing department. Thereafter, the researcher conducted non-face-to-face interviews in accordance with COVID-19 response guidelines. Additionally, before obtaining the consent form, he met each participant one-on-one and explained the research.

The interview was conducted at the time promised in a place where the interview could be kept confidential, such as a quiet place for non-face-to-face interviews. Based on the main questions of the interview guide, which were written in advance, additional questions were asked if necessary so that the research participants could fully talk about their experiences. Participant cards with information on the participants were created and filled out before the interview, which lasted approximately an hour. When the interview began, the participants were notified of the start and were thereafter recorded. Parts of the interview that were difficult to understand were clarified by the researcher asking additional questions at the end of the session. When it was determined that the group interview did not yield any new content and had reached saturation, the data collection was terminated.

The interview questions were in five formats: starting, introduction, transition, main, and closing questions [18]. Additionally, the questions were verified by two nurses in their 10th year of experience as to the validity of the contents of the interview. First, at the start of the interview, the interviewer softened the atmosphere through everyday conversation. Using a semi-structured questionnaire, the interview was started with the following introductory open question: "What comes to your mind when you think of therapeutic communication?". The transition question was, "What has been your experience in therapeutic communication with patients?". The main questions were, "What difficulties did you experience in therapeutic communication with patients in clinical practice?", "What qualities do you think nurses should possess for therapeutic communication?", and "What effects do nurses have on clinical communication?". These were followed by, "What education do you think is necessary for nurses in relation to therapeutic communication promotion?", and the closing question, "We discussed therapeutic communication promotion in clinical practice; is there anything else you want to say?".

The interview was conducted by asking a series of questions based on the participants' answers. The data were transcribed immediately after the interview by the co-researcher in the participants' language, and the responsible researcher checked the recorded data and confirmed the final transcript. All personal information of the participants was anonymized by numbering.

2.4. Data Analysis

The collected data were analyzed according to the phenomenological method of Colaizzi [17]. First, after repeatedly reading the transcribed data, the researcher identified the participants' experiences as well as their overall meanings, contents, and tones. Second, meaningful statements (words, phrases, and sentences) were extracted from the transcribed interview contents. Third, the researchers exchanged opinions on and extracted the common elements of the derived statements. Fourth, the meaning of the derived statements was re-stated in the researcher's language. Fifth, themes encompassing the entire experience were selected from the constructed meaning. Sixth, the meaning was reaffirmed by reviewing the data, and based on the derived subjects, it was categorized into theme clusters. Finally, after classifying the derived meanings and repeatedly sharing opinions, the structure and collection of the final categories were created. After verifying reliability and validity, the essential structure of the research phenomenon was described collectively.

2.5. Preparation of Researchers and Feasibility of Research

The responsible researcher has completed the development of nursing theory and qualitative research methodology in a doctoral course to lay the foundation for the theory and practice of qualitative research. Additionally, to expand the understanding of phenomenological research methods, efforts were made to elucidate the nature of the phenomenon by reading books related to phenomenology and qualitative research papers. Furthermore, all researchers tried to exclude their preconceptions as much as possible in order to have a neutral attitude during the study.

To secure the validity of the study, we followed the truth value, applicability, consistency, and neutrality criteria by Lincoln and Guba [19]. To secure the truth value, the recorded data were transcribed by the researcher and research assistant while listening to the recorded file. The recorded data were compared with the transcribed data while listening repeatedly two or more times. To secure applicability, two clinical nurses who were not participants in the study but had nursing experience with patients in similar situations were consulted. We intended to secure the consistency of data analysis by receiving feedback on the concepts and categories from two nursing professors with qualitative research experience. To secure neutrality, the research was conducted by excluding prejudice as much as possible.

2.6. Ethical Considerations

This study was conducted after obtaining approval from the Institutional Ethics and Life Committee of the Catholic University of Seoul Medical Center (approval number: KC21EASI0657). To guarantee the autonomy of the participants, the purpose and research method of the study were explained to them before the interview; additionally, written consent was obtained after explaining that they could withdraw their participation at any time. To ensure anonymity in the analysis process, the data were stored under numbers instead of participants' names.

3. Results

As a result of analyzing the interview data of the study participants, 22 themes, 14 theme clusters, and 5 category collections with more comprehensive meanings were extracted. The categories that were derived and analyzed are: "acquiring core competencies as nursing professionals", "improving patient-centered nursing performance", "forming a partnership treatment relationship", "obtaining clinical performance skills to solve problems", and "preparing efficient system improvement" (Table 2).

Table 2. Categories, theme clusters, and themes of therapeutic communication experiences of nurses caring for patients with hematology.

Themes	Theme Clusters	Categories
. Understanding from a patient's perspective based on values. Have an active response to the needs of the nurse	Empathize and take a proactive attitude from the patient's perspective	Acquiring core competencies as nursing professionals
. Feel rewarded in a comfortable atmosphere. Build self-efficacy by helping patients	Improve satisfaction and self-efficacy through work	
. Feeling a reaction to separate emotions in an emotional situation	Staying centered so that nurses do not get carried away	
. Patient-centered treatment for positive effects	Promote active patient engagement	Improving patient-centered nursing performance
. Active expression of nursing needs. Creating a sympathetic atmosphere in tense situations	Relieve anxiety through rapport formation	
. Improving trust in nurses by providing professional practical skills and knowledge	Increase confidence in nurses' work	
. Building a consensus on the idea of caring for family. Provide stability in the first hospital stay	Empathize and listen to the patient at their level	Forming a partnership treatment relationship
. Providing nursing care with respect for patients as people	Respect for the patient as a human being	
. Positive synergy effect in busy nursing situations. Patients affected by nurse behavior	Patient–nurse interaction	
. Self-development through the acquisition of professional knowledge and skills	Self-development	Obtain clinical performance skills to solve problems
. Feeling the need to provide educational opportunities according to communication and circumstances.. Expressing communication difficulties in different situations	Provide indirect experience opportunities for contextual scenarios	
. Adjusting the number of patients for the realization of full-time nursing. Difficulty in nursing work with increased severity	Efficient operation of nursing staff	Preparing efficient system improvement
. Sharing effective communication methods in different situations	Share experiences to improve nursing quality	
. Sharing information with other departments for patient care	Cooperate with other departments	

3.1. Category 1: Acquiring Core Competencies as Nursing Professionals

Participants stated that to communicate therapeutically with patients, they require certain core competencies as nursing professionals. They said that nurses should first approach the patient with an empathic and proactive attitude and that job satisfaction and self-efficacy increase through their practical work. Furthermore, they considered it important to have an attitude of not getting swayed by emotions during an emergency.

3.1.1. Empathize and Take a Proactive Attitude from the Patient's Perspective

The participants of this study agreed that therapeutic communication should be understood from the patient's perspective based on their values. Additionally, they considered that the patient's treatment effect would improve if they had sufficient time to initially approach and sympathize with the patient as medical staff.

> "I think communication involves knowing my values first, to empathize from the patient's point of view, and to understand the patient in an open manner" (Participant 11)

> "Many people suffer from mental illness as well as physical illness, and the more time we spend in sympathizing, asking, and listening first, the more effective it will be to treat patients" (Participant 4)

In this study, nurses said that they should have a proactive response or resolution to the patient's complaints. To communicate therapeutically, participants stated they should first be able to quickly recognize the symptoms that the patient complains about. Further, nurses should improve their treatment ability to solve nursing problems, which should be followed by therapeutic communication. One participant reported that a patient expressed gratitude for a quick response.

> "When I look at the patient's needs, I think I need an attitude of active participation" (Participant 17)

> "I think I can quickly recognize the symptoms that the patient complains of, solve the nursing problem, and then have smooth therapeutic communication if empathy and listening skills are added" (Participant 8)

> "While going through the morning rounds, we get caught up on the parts that we couldn't see and lacked, and when immediate treatment is provided, they trust us more and say 'thank you' later" (Participant 3)

3.1.2. Improve Satisfaction and Self-Efficacy through Work

The participants of this study said that it felt rewarding to communicate with patients in a comfortable atmosphere. Additionally, through therapeutic communication with patients, the nurses' work satisfaction increased when patients opened up.

> "Through therapeutic communication, nurses gain a lot of confidence in their nursing behavior, and their satisfaction with the nursing job increases, improving their efficiency in nursing" (Participant 9)

> "When I communicate therapeutically, I feel proud as a nurse and my job satisfaction increases when the patient opens up" (Participant 7)

> "I also feel that my satisfaction increases when I communicate with patients, and I perform my work with a more proactive attitude" (Participant 6)

The nurses stated that their self-efficacy was formed by helping patients and that their self-efficacy increased through therapeutic communication as the patients appeared to be emotionally stable.

> "I think my self-efficacy increases a lot because I can also help patients with their emotions" (Participant 18)

> "I think healing communication increases my self-efficacy and confidence in my work makes me better at therapeutic communication with patients. By doing this, it was good when the patient looked a little stable and expressed gratitude when I empathized with their feelings" (Participant 17)

3.1.3. Staying Centered So That Nurses Do Not Get Carried Away

In this study, the participants indicated that it is important to separate emotions from patients and maintain them consistently without overindulgence in emotional situations. Furthermore, they did not react emotionally when a patient's complaint came at a busy time.

> "There are a lot of patients dying. Therefore, I think it is necessary to control your mind to keep your emotions consistent without becoming overly immersed" (Participant 18)

> "I was having a difficult time adjusting [to] a room with the staff and coordinator of the hospital room because of a problem, and one patient was severely complaining. At that time, I treated the patient calmly rather than with anger. Nurses get hurt a lot, too. I'm dealing with these patients. Experiences that are not influenced by emotions are important" (Participant 2)

3.2. Category 2: Improving Patient-Centered Nursing Performance

Participants said that patient-centered nursing performance should be improved to communicate therapeutically with patients. Moreover, it is important to actively motivate patients to participate in their treatment, relieve their anxiety through rapport formation, and improve the trust in nurses.

3.2.1. Promote Active Patient Engagement

In this study, the participants reported that positive effects could be realized through patient-centered treatment. At first, patients might have tried to reject it, but if the nurses actively participated with the patient, they could later see the patients participating in their own treatments.

> "If patients actively participate in self-treatment and brush their teeth, gargle, and perform hand hygiene on their own, it will have a positive effect on preventing infection and recovering mucosal inflammation" (Participant 2)

> "In the case of bedridden patients, although they lie still and do nothing, they actively participate in the treatment. At first, [he] couldn't brush [his] teeth, but when I told him and wiped his face, the patient said he would wash his face and wash himself later. This support from medical personnel seems to provide patients with a sense of self-efficacy" (Participant 3)

3.2.2. Relieving Anxiety through Rapport Formation

In this study, the participants reported that it was possible to relieve patient anxiety by encouraging an active expression of nursing needs. Patients express their anxiety while forming a rapport with the nurse, and they are able to resolve their anxiety based on the nurse's listening and empathy.

> "If you express exactly what the patient wants through rapport formation, it seems to be more effective in treatment of and relieving the patient's anxiety" (Participant 5)

> "I believe patients' anxiety is reduced through therapeutic communication" (Participant 5)

> "When a patient expresses their feelings and condition to a nurse, the anxiety is relieved just by expressing it, and the nurse's empathy and listening can form a rapport, bond, and give credibility" (Participant 10)

In this study, the participants said that patient anxiety could be reduced by creating an empathetic atmosphere in a tense situation. They further reported that there was another way to relieve patients' anxiety with the help of other departments.

"A patient couldn't sleep at all on the day of the transplant because of anxiety. When I asked him if he slept well in the morning, he said he didn't sleep at all. So, I sympathized with the patient's situation by saying, 'Usually, the experience of treatment can come to mind and [patients] think a lot the day before the transplant'" (Participant 15)

"He was very depressed and anxious. He had some mental health problem, but he was a patient who refused to take medication. Nurses, of course, continued to listen to the patient with empathy, but through several interviews with the nun at the hospital, the patient's anxiety was reduced and mind was opened, so they could take prescribed drugs well" (Participant 11)

3.2.3. Increased Confidence in Nursing Work

This study's participants indicated that trust in nurses could be improved by providing professional practical skills and knowledge. The participants said that they had the expertise and an open attitude toward communicating therapeutically with patients to improve trust.

"I think providing nursing through practical skills and knowledge can improve patients' trust" (Participant 8)

"Above all, nurses need to have expertise in building trust. Basically, if you accept and communicate with the patient in an open manner with professional nursing knowledge, a trust relationship seems to form naturally" (Participant 11)

"When patients trust nurses through therapeutic communication, they seem to be better able to fulfill what they have to do on their own" (Participant 8)

3.3. Category 3: Forming a Partnership Treatment Relationship

In this study, the nurses said that a partnership treatment relationship should be formed to communicate therapeutically with patients. The participants said that they could sympathize and listen to the patients at their level and form a partnership treatment relationship by respecting patients as human beings and the interaction between patients and nurses.

3.3.1. Empathize and Listen to the Patient at Their Level

In this study, the participants considered it necessary to sympathize and listen to individual patient cases. They said it was important to form a consensus through an attitude of caring for the family. Additionally, nursing from the patient's point of view should be considered.

"I think empathy is what nurses need the most. Most of the time, I care for older people, so if you're my mother . . . If it's my dad . . . 'I'm going to nurse him like this'" (Participant 4)

"Nurses are busy at work, but I think nursing should be done based on the attitude of empathizing and listening to patients" (Participant 6)

Further, participants reported that it was necessary to provide stability when a patient stays in the hospital for the first time. The nurses said that they provided therapeutic communication by providing necessary information to patients staying in the hospital for the first time based on their clinical experience.

"In some cases, children are diagnosed with leukemia because they think it's just a cold, and in others, their guardians usually blame themselves. In that case, they say, 'It's not the guardian's fault,' and they can treat it. It was good when I said, 'If you show the patient how you overcome it together, and not the mother having a hard time'" (Participant 13)

"When I provide information based on my clinical experience to patients who come to the hospital and have been diagnosed for the first time, I feel like I am communicating therapeutically" (Participant 9)

3.3.2. Respect for the Patient as a Human Being

The participants said that it is necessary to provide nursing care by respecting patients as humans and that through therapeutic communication with patients, they understand and sympathize more with the patient as a person.

"I think we need to look at the patient as a person, ask how he feels today, and whether he is in a better condition than yesterday, and ask them questions that allow them to be seen as a person and not a patient" (Participant 10)

"It felt like I was understanding, empathizing, and communicating with patients in different situations in a therapeutic way. I think my personal side is also developing" (Participant 19)

3.3.3. Patient–Nurse Interaction

In this study, we found that a positive synergy effect occurred due to the interaction between patients and nurses. Participants said that it was particularly effective in a busy nursing environment.

"When I communicate therapeutically with patients, I feel like I'm gaining strength and healing. It's therapeutic communication for patients, and I think sometimes I try to communicate to gain strength, and I tend to take care of patients. So, in the end, when the patient and the nurse really communicate, I think they're treating each other" (Participant 1). "I think it's important that we look at the patient's condition first and ask questions while we're rounding to make him feel that he's getting attention. The patient also seems to have an effect on the treatment effect by telling them about their uncomfortable situations first" (Participant 13)

In this study, the nurses reported that patients were affected by nurses' behaviors.

"I think every nurse's behavior affects the interaction relationship with the patient" (Participant 3)

"I think it is also important to allow nurses and patients to work together to solve patient health problems" (Participant 3)

3.4. Category 4: Obtain Clinical Performance Skills to Solve Problems

The participants reported that to achieve therapeutic communication skills, a clinical performance ability for problem-solving should be acquired. For this purpose, nurses should develop themselves and provide an opportunity for self-development for problem-solving and scenarios on how to cope in a similar situation.

3.4.1. Self-Development

The participants stated that self-development should be achieved through the acquisition of professional knowledge and skills. Moreover, accurate information delivery and continuous studying are necessary for therapeutic communication.

"As a nurse, I think that such professional knowledge and skills should be the basis, and then communication skills should be included" (Participant 7)

"I had a difficult time when I was intimidated because I didn't know the answer when a patient asked me a question. I think it is necessary to study the disease continuously. That way, I think I will be able to communicate therapeutically with the patient, gain confidence, and have an attitude of listening" (Participant 12)

Nurses in this study said that the ability to determine and solve nursing needs based on priorities is necessary. Having the ability to resolve a patient's symptoms is also a method of therapeutic communication.

"I think accurate care for the nursing problems that patients require should be given first. I think it is more effective to control pain first in patients who are sick and then to communicate therapeutically. I also think the nursing ability to identify and respond to the patient's needs first is necessary" (Participant 20)

"For therapeutic communication, I think we need the ability to solve the symptoms that the patient complains of first. There was a patient who had delusions of damage or delirium during the transplant and was restless because he couldn't sleep. We listened first to the constant appeals and complaints, and then consulted with the doctor to add drugs and allow the caregiver to stay stable" (Participant 3)

3.4.2. Provide Indirect Experience Opportunities for Contextual Scenarios

The participants of this study said that they felt the need to receive educational opportunities depending on the situation and that they wanted to communicate effectively with patients by receiving education on how to communicate with them.

"I think we need an education program that teaches us how to listen and respond when talking to patients" (Participant 13)

"I've taken communication education at a hospital, and I don't think it's often, but I hope there's a regular one" (Participant 15)

In the group interview, difficulty in communicating according to various situations was expressed. Participants reported that they felt awkward and worried when communicating with patients. Therefore, there were several demands for education on how to communicate based on certain situations.

"To be honest, it's very hard for me to start talking. For example, if you are a guardian of new patients and you are crying, or if the guardian is having a hard time due to the death of the patient, it would be good to receive training on how to start conversation and what words are helpful to the other person" (Participant 10)

"There's a patient who doesn't say a word. In such a situation, I am worried about how to approach and how to open my heart" (Participant 4)

3.5. Category 5: Preparing Efficient System Improvement

The group interview revealed that the efficient hospital system should be improved to communicate therapeutically with patients. Participants said that they should streamline the operations of nursing personnel, share experiences to improve the quality of nursing, and cooperate with other departments.

3.5.1. Efficient Operation of Nursing Staff

Participants reported that the number of patients a nurse is in charge of should be adjusted according to the patients' symptom severity. They added that it was necessary to adjust the number of patients for full-time nursing, indicating that the number of assigned patients at work was large and there were cases where they wanted to communicate therapeutically with one patient but became frustrated because it did not go as intended.

"If the number of patients in charge per nurse is low, I think we can provide more full-time care to each patient" (Participant 8)

"My work is so busy, and I'm overwhelmed with work that I can't afford it myself. I want to communicate therapeutically with the patient, but sometimes I wonder if they are serious about it" (Participant 18)

In this study, the participants expressed that nursing work is difficult with increased severity. Further, they stated that when they see patients with hematology, they are pressed for work and time and are thus unable to respond suitably; if they are supplemented with more manpower, they will have sufficient time to conduct better therapeutic communication.

"There are so many symptoms that patients with hematology complain of, and the severity is high; so, I think it is necessary to make efforts to reduce the number of patients per nurse" (Participant 6)

"I think we can better communicate the therapeutic communication we want to only when we replenish the nursing workforce so that I can have time for the patient as well" (Participant 5)

"On days when I come to work as an over-member, I think I can definitely listen to patients more and take care of even the smallest things for them, so I can communicate well in therapy" (Participant 2)

3.5.2. Share Experiences to Improve Nursing Quality

In this study, effective communication methods were shared according to the situation. Participants expressed their desire to communicate effectively with patients by sharing other people's experiences.

"I think it's very important to communicate about situations that a patient may experience such as discomfort and dying conditions. Even if it's not a simulation, I think it's better for more experienced people to share how to communicate in such a situation" (Participant 5)

3.5.3. Cooperation with Other Departments

In this study, the nurses said they tried to share information with other departments regarding patient treatment. They said that they would be able to identify enough patients by sharing the parts of the treatments that they did not know about while nursing and communicating therapeutically based on the patients' conditions.

"I think it is necessary to promote communication with other medical staff. If we share the patient's treatment plan that the doctors' team is thinking about, and what the nurse does not know, such as what we discussed with the rehabilitation and social work teams, we will be able to know the patient's condition well and nurse accordingly" (Participant 10)

4. Discussion

This study was conducted to explore the therapeutic communication experiences of nurses caring for patients with hematology. As a result of an analysis using Colaizzi's [17] phenomenological method, 5 categories and 14 theme clusters were derived from the data. The five categories were "acquiring core competencies as nursing professionals", "improving patient-centered nursing performance", "forming a partnership treatment relationship", "obtaining clinical performance skills to solve problems", and "preparing efficient system improvement".

In the category of "acquiring core competencies as nursing professionals", the themes were: "empathize and take a proactive attitude from the patient's perspective", "improve satisfaction and self-efficacy through work", and "stay centered so that nurses do not get carried away". This category revealed that nurses approach nursing from the patient's perspective and improve their self-efficacy through work, indicating that emotions during nursing work should be separated from professional skills. The finding of nurses gaining understanding through the patients' viewpoint based on their values was similar to a study that said therapeutic communication skills such as reflection, empathy, and listening were necessary for an effective therapeutic relationship [20]. The present participants expressed that their self-efficacy was formed by helping patients, and it was necessary to isolate their emotions during emotional situations. This is similar to a previous study that reported that nurse job satisfaction, work commitment, self-efficacy, self-regulation, and prediction technology development increase patient satisfaction [21]. Additionally, emotional distancing can result in providing the best care to patients while protecting the mental health of nurses, which helps to reduce nurses' emotional labor and maintain professionalism [22].

However, there is insufficient institutional supplementation or education for nurses regarding separating emotions or inculcating empathy for patients in hospitals. Therefore, to acquire core competencies as a professional nurse, it is necessary to not only improve the nurse's active response method to patients and the rewarding feeling when caring for patients but also to support nurses in not becoming overwhelmed by their emotions.

In the category of "improving patient-centered nursing performance", the derived themes were: "promote active patient engagement", "relieving anxiety through rapport formation" and "increased confidence in nursing work". In this category, the patient's active participation in treatments showed a positive effect, and communication from the patient's perspective resulted in reduced anxiety.

This indicates that confidence-building between patients and nurses allows patients to communicate freely [23]. Moreover, confidence-building serves as the basis for a therapeutic relationship and allows patients to respect and comply with the nurse's judgment [20]. Furthermore, nurses reported that patients' confidence in nurses improved through the utilization of practical skills and knowledge, and prior results show that patients can obtain necessary medical information through communication with nurses while improving treatment performance and health management [24].

In recent studies, patient participation in the medical system is a legal right, requiring patients to participate in decisions related to their healthcare planning, effectiveness, and evaluation [25]. It has been reported that the concept of patient-centeredness is important in providing integrated treatment [26]. Therefore, for therapeutic communication, patients should actively participate in treatment, and nurses should provide patients with opportunities to express their nursing needs.

Additionally, nurses need to make individual efforts to improve standard practical skills and proficiency in work to improve professionalism.

In the category of "forming a partnership treatment relationship", the derived themes were: "empathize and listen to the patient at their level", "respect for the patient as a human being", and "patient–nurse interaction". In this category, it was found that nursing care should be provided with respect to the patient as a person and with an attitude of caring to the family. In addition, even during busy nursing situations, the interactions between a patient and a nurse may have a positive effect, and the patient may be affected by the nurse's behavior. This is in line with previous studies that have reported that therapeutic communication can be a small spark that generates strong energy and clarifies the aims pursued by the nurse and the patient [24]. The patient's response may vary depending on the characteristics of the interaction, including the communication used by the nurse [27]. Therefore, for therapeutic communication, the nurse pays more attention to the patient and communicates directly to empathize with the patient's pain [28]. However, research on the interaction between patients and nurses is insufficient [25,27]. Therefore, further research on the interaction between patients and nurses is required.

In the category of "obtaining clinical performance skills to solve problems", the derived themes were: "self-development" and "provide indirect experience opportunities for contextual scenarios". In this category, the necessity of providing educational opportunities for nurses appeared to be due to self-development through the acquisition of professional knowledge and skills and experiencing difficulties in communication in various situations. It is important to understand how nurses continue to improve their professionalism as their knowledge expands and expectations for better outcomes increase in an era of increasing demand for accountability in healthcare [29]. Similar to previous studies [24], the development of educational programs and effectiveness verification studies is necessary to promote therapeutic communication. In today's technical and complex medical environment, the educational level and years of experience of nurses are important not only for them to continue providing effective care but also for their expectations regarding lifelong learning [29].

In the category of "preparing efficient system improvement", the derived themes were: "efficient operation of nursing staff", "share experiences to improve nursing quality", and "cooperation with other departments". This category highlights the need to adjust the number of patients for the realization of full-time nursing and to adjust the number of nurses according to the patient's increased symptom severity. In addition, it is important to provide nurses with opportunities to share effective communication methods based on individual situations, along with sharing information with other departments for patient treatment. This indicates that patients want nurses to spend more time helping them solve problems [30]. Due to lack of time, nurses may ask superficial questions during interviews, making patients feel the impatience of the nurses, especially in the case of new nurses who are pressed for time, with patients considering it useless to talk to nurses as they appear busy [24]. Nursing in oncology particularly requires innovative recruitment strategies, onboarding and continuous education programs, industrial safety measures, and antiburn interventions as nurses are scarce, and there are recruitment barriers (e.g., awareness of demanding specialties with complex treatments and dangerous work environments) and burnout [31]. Therefore, it is critical to provide institutional support for nurses to self-develop through the acquisition of professional knowledge and skills and to provide indirect experience opportunities through the development of situation-specific scenarios. Additionally, it is necessary to systematically provide opportunities for communication by connecting experienced nurses with new nurses to educate them on effective communication according to different situations. Furthermore, interaction and teamwork between experts are important, and cultural conditions and contextual determinants should be included at this time [32]. Moreover, sufficient knowledge of each other's work, a culture of mutual respect, the recognition of each other's expertise and capabilities, and free and open information exchange are necessary, in addition to sufficient time and resources for establishing effective and continuous relationships between care providers [33,34].

As shown by previous studies, organizational system design is needed to foster better partnerships and information sharing and to support integration between providers, healthcare professionals, and patients [33]. Further, it will be necessary to improve the system for sharing information with other departments for the more efficient treatment of patients. Nurses are the best professionals to coordinate patients' care because they spend more time with patients than any other healthcare professional [31]. In particular, hematology nurses should be able to form appropriate therapeutic communication with patients by sensitively examining the patient's condition, which can change rapidly depending on the progression of the disease. However, nurses who take care of patients with hematology in a clinical setting see many patients and are, thus, in a hurry to perform nursing tasks rather than conduct therapeutic communication. Additionally, when caring for patients with hematology in clinical settings, although the nurses know that therapeutic communication is necessary, they may not know the appropriate method, hence experiencing difficulties and raising the demand for therapeutic communication education and training. Therefore, for nurses to effectively communicate therapeutically with patients with hematology, it is necessary to train them in various approaches while considering the patient's symptoms and emotions [24].

The limitations of this study are as follows. First, it was difficult to confirm whether therapeutic communication was conducted in accordance with the stage and disease type of patients with hematology. Second, the findings of this study should be generalized with caution as the research results were obtained from a single institution. Third, the average experience of caring for patients with hematology was four years and eight months, and it was difficult to confirm whether there was a gap in therapeutic communication quality.

This study is meaningful in that it is the first to examine the therapeutic communication experience of nurses caring for patients with hematological cancer. Additionally, this study does not represent a specific sample, and the data and results of this study can help new nurses in providing care to patients with hematological cancer.

5. Conclusions

In this study, a focus group interview was conducted and analyzed using a phenomenological method to gain an in-depth understanding of the therapeutic communication experiences of nurses caring for patients with hematological cancer. It was confirmed that the nurses possessed core competencies for conducting therapeutic communication as nursing professionals, formed partnerships at the patient center, acquired clinical performance capabilities, and implemented efficient institutional improvements to solve problems. This study's findings can enable the provision of high-quality nursing to patients by improving the therapeutic communication ability of nurses caring for patients with hematological cancer. In addition, the findings can be used as basic data for the development of a therapeutic communication program through the interactions between patients and nurses. Additionally, based on the results of this study, follow-up research should develop a standardized tool that can measure therapeutic communication ability. Moreover, based on the theory, it is necessary to develop a therapeutic communication promotion program for nurses caring for patients with hematology cancer.

Author Contributions: H.-J.L.: conceptualization, methodology, formal analysis, investigation, writing—original draft, writing—review and editing, visualization, supervision; B.-M.P.: conceptualization, methodology, formal analysis, writing—original draft, writing—review and editing, visualization, supervision; M.-J.S.: investigation; D.-Y.K.: investigation. All authors have read and agreed to the published version of the manuscript.

Funding: This research received no external funding.

Institutional Review Board statement: This study was conducted according to the guidelines of the Declaration of Helsinki and approved by the Institutional Review Board of the affiliated institution (KC21EASI0657; date of approval: 28 December 2021) in Seoul, Republic of Korea.

Informed Consent statement: Not applicable.

Data Availability Statement: Not applicable.

Conflicts of Interest: The authors have no conflict of interest to declare.

References

1. Fleischer, S.; Berg, A.; Zimmermann, M.; Wüste, K.; Behrens, J. Nurse-patient interaction and communication: A systematic literature review. *J. Public Health* **2009**, *17*, 339–353. [CrossRef]
2. Maame Kissiwaa Amoah, V.; Anokye, R.; Boakye, D.S.; Gyamfi, N. Perceived barriers to effective therapeutic communication among nurses and patients at Kumasi South Hospital. *Cogent Med.* **2018**, *5*, 1459341. [CrossRef]
3. Sharma, N.; Gupta, V. Therapeutic communication. In *StatPearls*; StatPearls Publishing LLC: Tampa, FL, USA, 2022.
4. Fite, R.O.; Assefa, M.; Demissie, A.; Belachew, T. Predictors of therapeutic communication between nurses and hospitalized patients. *Heliyon* **2019**, *5*, e02665. [CrossRef]
5. Granados-Gámez, G.; Sáez-Ruiz, I.M.; Márquez-Hernández, V.V.; Rodríguez-García, M.; Aguilera-Manrique, G.; Cibanal-Juan, M.L.; Gutiérrez-Puertas, L. Development and validation of the questionnaire to analyze the communication of nurses in nurse-patient therapeutic communication. *Patient Educ. Couns.* **2022**, *105*, 145–150. [CrossRef]
6. Granados-Gámez, G.; Sáez-Ruiz, I.M.; Márquez-Hernández, V.V.; Ybarra-Sagarduy, J.L.; Aguilera-Manrique, G.; Gutiérrez-Puertas, L. Systematic review of measurement properties of self-reported instruments for evaluating therapeutic communication. *West. J. Nurs. Res.* **2021**, *43*, 791–804. [CrossRef]
7. Negi, S.; Kaur, H.; Singh, G.M.; Pugazhendi, S. Quality of nurse patient therapeutic communication and overall patient satisfaction during their hospitalization stay. *Int. J. Med. Sci. Public Health* **2017**, *6*, 675–679. [CrossRef]

8. Amoah, V.M.K.; Anokye, R.; Boakye, D.S.; Acheampong, E.; Budu-Ainooson, A.; Okyere, E.; Kumi-Boateng, G.; Yeboah, C.; Afriyie, J.O. A qualitative assessment of perceived barriers to effective therapeutic communication among nurses and patients. *BMC Nurs.* **2019**, *18*, 4. [CrossRef]
9. Das Mohamed, D.A.; Ahmed, D.A.M. Effect of nurse's therapeutic communication and protecting patient's rights on patient's satisfaction. *Tanta Sci. Nurs. J.* **2019**, *16*, 113–132. [CrossRef]
10. Han, J.; Liu, J.-E.; Zheng, X.-L.; Ma, Y.-H.; Xiao, Q.; Ding, Y.-M. Caring in nursing: Investigating the meaning of caring from the perspective of Chinese children living with leukemia. *Int. J. Nurs. Sci.* **2014**, *1*, 34–41. [CrossRef]
11. Geres, H.; Kotchetkov, R. Nursing in patients with hematological malignancies. *Int. J. Hematol. Oncol.* **2020**, *9*. [CrossRef]
12. Citak, E.A.; Toruner, E.K.; Gunes, N.B. Exploring communication difficulties in pediatric hematology: Oncology nurses. *Asian Pac. J. Cancer Prev.* **2013**, *14*, 5477–5482. [CrossRef] [PubMed]
13. McCarthy, B.; O'Donovan, M.; Trace, A. A new therapeutic communication model "TAGEET" to help nurses engage therapeutically with patients suspected of or confirmed with COVID-19. *J. Clin. Nurs.* **2021**, *30*, 1184–1191. [CrossRef] [PubMed]
14. Park, K.O. Nurses' experience of health communication with doctors in the clinical fields. *J. Korean Acad. Nurs. Adm.* **2015**, *21*, 53–63. [CrossRef]
15. Pehrson, C.; Banerjee, S.C.; Manna, R.; Shen, M.J.; Hammonds, S.; Coyle, N.; Krueger, C.A.; Maloney, E.; Zaider, T.; Bylund, C.L. Responding empathically to patients: Development, implementation, and evaluation of a communication skills training module for oncology nurses. *Patient Educ. Couns.* **2016**, *99*, 610–616. [CrossRef]
16. Bauer, M.W.; Gaskell, G. *Qualitative Researching With Text, Image and Sound: A Practical Handbook for Social Research*; Sage: Newbury Park, CA, USA, 2000.
17. Colaizzi, P.F. Psychological research as the phenomenologist views it. In *Existential-Phenomenological Alternatives for Psychology*; Valle, R.S., King, M., Eds.; Oxford University Press: Oxford, UK, 1978; p. 6.
18. Krueger, R.A. *Focus Groups: A Practical Guide for Applied Research*; Sage Publications: Newbury Park, CA, USA, 2014.
19. Guba, E.G.; Lincoln, Y.S. *Effective Evaluation: Improving the Usefulness of Evaluation Results through Responsive and Naturalistic Approaches*; Jossey-Bass: San Francisco, CA, USA, 1981.
20. Kang, P.; Kang, J. Nurses' experience with inpatients in comprehensive nursing care service: A phenomenological approach. *J. Korean Acad. Nurs. Adm.* **2021**, *27*, 149–158. [CrossRef]
21. De Simone, S.; Planta, A.; Cicotto, G. The role of job satisfaction, work engagement, self-efficacy and agentic capacities on nurses' turnover intention and patient satisfaction. *Appl. Nurs. Res.* **2018**, *39*, 130–140. [CrossRef]
22. Kim, J.; Kim, S.; Byun, M. Emotional distancing in nursing: A concept analysis. *Nurs. Forum.* **2020**, *55*, 595–602. [CrossRef]
23. Buelow, J.; Miller, W.; Fishman, J. Development of an epilepsy nursing communication tool: Improving the quality of interactions Between nurses and patients with seizures. *J. Neurosci. Nurs.* **2018**, *50*, 74–80. [CrossRef]
24. Joung, J.; Park, Y. Exploring the therapeutic communication practical experience of mental health nurses. *J. Korean Acad. Psychiatr. Ment. Health Nurs.* **2019**, *28*, 321–332. [CrossRef]
25. Park, B.M. Development and effect of a fall prevention program based on King's theory of goal attainment in long-term care hospitals: An experimental study. *Healthcare* **2021**, *9*, 715. [CrossRef]
26. Singer, S.J.; Burgers, J.; Friedberg, M.; Rosenthal, M.B.; Leape, L.; Schneider, E. Defining and measuring integrated patient care: Promoting the next frontier in health care delivery. *Med. Care Res. Rev.* **2011**, *68*, 112–127. [CrossRef] [PubMed]
27. Kim, E.J. Nurse-patient interaction patterns and patient satisfaction in the emergency department. *J. Korean Acad. Nurs.* **2010**, *40*, 99–109. [CrossRef] [PubMed]
28. Lee, E.; Chang, S.S. Factors influencing depression of nurses among comprehensive nursing care service ward. *Korean J. Occup. Health Nurs.* **2016**, *25*, 340–351. [CrossRef]
29. Bathish, M.; Wilson, C.; Potempa, K. Deliberate practice and nurse competence. *Appl. Nurs. Res.* **2018**, *40*, 106–109. [CrossRef] [PubMed]
30. McLaughlin, C. An exploration of psychiatric nurses' and patients' opinions regarding in-patient care for suicidal patients. *J. Adv. Nurs.* **1999**, *29*, 1042–1051. [CrossRef]
31. Challinor, J.M.; Alqudimat, M.R.; Teixeira, T.O.A.; Oldenmenger, W.H. Oncology nursing workforce: Challenges, solutions, and future strategies. *Lancet Oncol.* **2020**, *21*, e564–e574. [CrossRef]
32. McCallin, A. Interdisciplinary practice–A matter of teamwork: An integrated literature review. *J. Clin. Nurs.* **2001**, *10*, 419–428. [CrossRef] [PubMed]
33. Steihaug, S.; Johannessen, A.K.; Ådnanes, M.; Paulsen, B.; Mannion, R. Challenges in achieving collaboration in clinical practice: The case of Norwegian health care. *Int. J. Integr. Care* **2016**, *16*, 3. [CrossRef]
34. Tsasis, P.; Evans, J.M.; Owen, S. Reframing the challenges to integrated care: A complex-adaptive systems perspective. *Int. J. Integr. Care* **2012**, *12*, e190. [CrossRef]

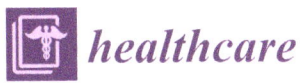

Article

Correlation between Quality of Life under Treatment and Current Life Satisfaction among Cancer Survivors Aged 75 Years and Older Receiving Outpatient Chemotherapy in Ishikawa Prefecture, Japan

Yoshiko Kitamura [1,*], Hisao Nakai [1], Tomoe Hashimoto [1], Yuko Morikawa [1] and Yoshiharu Motoo [2]

1 School of Nursing, Kanazawa Medical University, 1-1 Uchinada, Kahoku 920-0265, Ishikawa, Japan
2 Komatsu Sophia Hospital, Komatsu 923-0861, Ishikawa, Japan
* Correspondence: kitamu@kanazawa-med.ac.jp; Tel.: +81-76-286-2211 (ext.7568)

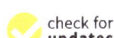

Citation: Kitamura, Y.; Nakai, H.; Hashimoto, T.; Morikawa, Y.; Motoo, Y. Correlation between Quality of Life under Treatment and Current Life Satisfaction among Cancer Survivors Aged 75 Years and Older Receiving Outpatient Chemotherapy in Ishikawa Prefecture, Japan. *Healthcare* 2022, *10*, 1863. https://doi.org/10.3390/healthcare10101863

Academic Editor: Qiuping Li

Received: 4 August 2022
Accepted: 16 September 2022
Published: 24 September 2022

Publisher's Note: MDPI stays neutral with regard to jurisdictional claims in published maps and institutional affiliations.

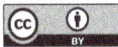

Copyright: © 2022 by the authors. Licensee MDPI, Basel, Switzerland. This article is an open access article distributed under the terms and conditions of the Creative Commons Attribution (CC BY) license (https://creativecommons.org/licenses/by/4.0/).

Abstract: Life satisfaction is increasingly important for older cancer survivors as the global population ages and the life expectancy 29 of cancer survivors increases. This study sought to identify factors associated with physical symptoms, quality of life under treatment, and current life satisfaction in cancer survivors aged 75 years and older receiving outpatient chemotherapy. Information about treatment for cancer survivors was collected from electronic medical records, and interviews were conducted to assess life satisfaction under treatment. Participants were older cancer survivors in Ishikawa, Japan. Of the participants, 80% lived on the Noto Peninsula. The average linear distance traveled for treatment was 40.7 km. The factors associated with patients' dissatisfaction with their current lives included general malaise (odds ratio: 9.61; 95% confidence interval: 1.28–72.22) and being less happy now than when they were younger (odds ratio: 10.559; 95% confidence interval: 1.50–74.24). In outpatient cancer treatment for survivors aged 75 years and older, support should consider the distance to the hospital. As in past studies, general malaise was shown to have a negative impact on the lives of cancer survivors aged 75 years or older. Support providers should pay attention to patients' general malaise when providing support.

Keywords: cancer survivors; chemotherapy; personal satisfaction; quality of life

1. Introduction

The number of cancer survivors continues to increase because of advances in early detection and treatment, in addition to the aging and growth of the population [1]. Estimates up to 2035 predict an increase in the number of older cancer patients worldwide [2]. In the United States, the number of older cancer survivors continues to increase, and effective interventions to address the complex needs of older cancer survivors are currently lacking [3]. Older cancer survivors often live with existing or developing comorbidities and have complex medical and psychosocial care needs [4,5].

The maintenance and improvement of physical function and health-related quality of life (QOL) in the treatment of older cancer survivors are increasingly regarded as hard endpoints for clinical cancer research [6]. Regarding QOL and happiness in older cancer survivors, a study of people aged 75 years and older in Sweden reported that people with cancer had lower QOL than people without cancer [7]. Older breast cancer survivors were found to have lower QOL than younger women, and comorbidities and socioeconomic status have also been reported to affect QOL [8]. Moreover, older breast cancer survivors are reported to have lower life satisfaction, mastery, and spiritual well-being than younger survivors [9]. Many studies of satisfaction among older cancer survivors have examined satisfaction with care and medical treatment. Cancer survivors who recognize that they are being treated with courtesy and respect by their providers [10] and are receiving adequate information and communication from providers have been shown to report greater satisfaction with health care [11–13].

Reports of QOL under treatment and life satisfaction of older cancer survivors [14] revealed that, among survivors aged 60 years and older, social support from friends and family is a predictive factor for social well-being [15]. Furthermore, health-related QOL for cancer survivors and their spouses or partners has been shown to affect satisfaction with cancer treatment outcomes [16]. Although population projections of global cancer patients by age group indicate an increase in the number of cancer patients aged 75 years and older [2], only a small number of studies have examined cancer survivors in this age group. For example, one study examined mental health in breast cancer survivors aged 65 years and older [17]. Approximately half of the participants in the study were aged 75 years and older, but they were not analyzed by age group [17]. In eastern Europe, relative survival rates for breast cancer were reported to decrease rapidly with age (75 years and older) [18]. Risk factors for psychosocial well-being and psychosocial problems in cancer survivors aged 65 years and older have been examined, but no analyses focusing on those aged 75 years and older have been reported [19]. Importantly, no previous studies have examined QOL under treatment or post-treatment symptoms among older cancer survivors aged 75 years and older while also examining factors related to life satisfaction.

Japan's population is aging at an unprecedented rate. Considering that the number of older people is predicted to continue to increase in Japan until 2036 [20] and that the life expectancy of cancer patients is improving [21], it is important to understand the symptoms that cancer survivors aged 75 years and older are living with, and the factors that affect their life satisfaction, to identify the most effective support to provide to them.

The purpose of the current study was to evaluate the correlation between physical symptoms and QOL under treatment of cancer patients aged 75 years and older receiving outpatient chemotherapy in Ishikawa Prefecture, Japan, and their current life satisfaction. By studying the physical symptoms and QOL under treatment of cancer survivors aged 75 years and older, and by identifying factors related to satisfaction with their current lives, it was possible to obtain survivors' suggestions for improving their QOL for the remainder of their lives. This report from Japan, in which population aging is progressing at a more rapid pace compared with that in the rest of the world, will serve as a reference for other countries in which population aging is receiving increasing attention.

2. Methods

2.1. Ethical Considerations

This research was conducted in accordance with the Declaration of Helsinki, 1995 (as revised in Seoul, 2008), and was carried out with the consent of the University Medical Research Ethics Review Committees at the authors' universities (No. I691). Prior to the interviews, we explained to participants, verbally and in writing, the purpose and significance of the study, the research method, that participation was voluntary, and that individuals would not be identified when the results are published.

2.2. Data Collection

We studied patients aged 75 years and older who were receiving outpatient chemotherapy at Kanazawa Medical University Hospital in Ishikawa Prefecture, Japan. Ishikawa Prefecture is located in the center of Hokuriku facing the Sea of Japan, with the Noto Peninsula in the north protruding into the Sea of Japan [22]. The population of Ishikawa Prefecture is approximately 1.12 million [23], and approximately 30% of the population is aged 65 years and older [24].

This study utilized a cross-sectional survey method. Data were collected through hospital medical records and interviews with participants. Interviews were conducted by two people: a research representative and a research collaborator. The research collaborator underwent interview training. We created an original questionnaire for this research. To explore the physical symptoms of older cancer survivors, we created questionnaire items by referencing common cancer and treatment-related symptoms listed by the National Cancer Center Japan [25]. Items from the Barthel Index [26,27] were used to examine the current activities of daily living. The Philadelphia Geriatric Center Morale Scale [28] and positive or negative feelings of morale [29] items were used to interview patients regarding overall satisfaction and current life satisfaction. The survey was conducted from 1 March to 6 April 2022.

2.3. Survey Details

Table 1 shows the survey items.

Table 1. Survey items.

Items obtained from hospital medical records
Background
Information included age, sex, municipality of residence, cancer site, time since cancer diagnosis, and presence or absence of metastases.
The frequency of visits
Response options were "every week", "every 2 weeks", "every 3 weeks", or "other".
Underlying diseases
Response options were diseases of the "circulatory system", "respiratory system", "cranial nerve system", "endocrine system", "renal/urinary system", "motor system", "sensory system", "other", and "none" (multiple answers allowed).
Past treatment according to treatment method
Response options were "surgery", "radiation therapy", "chemotherapy", and "other" (multiple answers allowed).
Medication status
This item was responded to as a "yes/no" question for "oral medications", "opioids", "non-opioids", "cancer therapeutic drugs", "sleeping pills", "hypertension medication", "diabetes drugs", and "laxatives".
Items for which participants were asked to report details
Annual income
Responses were classified into three categories: "less than 2.8 million yen", "between 2.8 million and 3.4 million yen", "3.4 million yen or more", and "I don't know" [30], referring to the self-pay ratio of long-term care insurance service charges in Japan.
Cancer insurance coverage
Responses were classified into three categories: "I have insurance", "I don't have insurance", and "I don't know".
Support providers
Participants responded in a "yes/no" format regarding "cohabitants (people who lived with them)", "relatives nearby", and "people who would rush to help in an emergency".
Physical symptoms
Responses included "general malaise", "loss of appetite", "pain", "constipation", "respiratory distress", and "other", which respondents reported using four options: "strongly present", "present", "slightly present", and "not present".
Activities of daily living
Responses included "I can go up and down the stairs", "prepare meals", "eat meals by myself", "bathe by myself", "urinate by myself", "defecate by myself", "change clothing by myself", and "straighten my posture by myself", and were classified into four categories: "independent", "need to be watched over", "partial assistance", and "total assistance".
Self-care behaviors
Responses included "being able to see a doctor at a designated date and time", "being able to go to the hospital by oneself", and "taking oral medicines as instructed", which were classified into four categories: "independent", "need to be watched over", "partial assistance", and "total assistance".

Table 1. Cont.

Satisfaction with life
"I started to worry about small things", "I think I'm happier now than when I was young", "I'm unable to sleep", "I get agitated easily", "I feel lonely", and "I feel uncomfortable with my family" were reported using four response options: "strongly agree", "agree", "disagree", and "strongly disagree".
Satisfaction with current life
Responses were classified using four response options: "strongly agree", "agree", "disagree", and "strongly disagree".

2.4. Analysis Methods

We analyzed the responses of participants who answered all of the following items: annual income, cancer insurance coverage, support providers, degree of current physical symptoms, activities of daily living, self-care behavior, and life satisfaction.

To understand participants' characteristics, the median and range deviations were calculated for age and time since their cancer diagnosis. We calculated the distribution of treatment history by frequency of hospital visits, underlying diseases, and treatment methods. We created a spider graph that connected a straight line from Kanazawa Medical University Hospital to the government office of the participants' residences and calculated the geographical distribution. ESRI ArcGIS Pro (ESRI; Redlands, CA, USA) was used to analyze geographic distribution.

To evaluate the factors affecting current life satisfaction, for age, the median age was used to categorize participants into two categories of below and above the age of 80. The median time since cancer diagnosis was used to categorize participants into two categories: under and over 17.5 months. Regarding annual income, 2.8 million yen (the base amount at which the self-pay ratio for long-term care insurance services in Japan goes from 10% to 20%) was used, with participants classified into the two categories of "2.8 million yen or above" and "less than 2.8 million yen or unknown", with the latter classified as "Other".

For cancer insurance coverage, "I have insurance" was classified as "Yes", and "I don't have insurance/I don't know" were classified as "Other". For the degree of physical symptoms, "many symptoms/symptoms present" was classified as "Yes" and "a few symptoms/no symptoms" were classified as "Other". For treatment response, "independent" was classified as "Independent" and "being watched over/partial assistance/total assistance" was classified as "Other". For life satisfaction, "strongly agree/agree" was classified as "Agree" and "disagree/strongly disagree" was classified as "Disagree".

The correlation between satisfaction with current life and basic attributes, annual income, cancer insurance coverage, support providers, time since cancer diagnosis, metastasis, underlying disease, medication status, degree of physical symptoms, self-care behavior, and life satisfaction were assessed using the Chi-square test or Fisher's exact test.

With satisfaction with current life as the dependent variable, a binary logistic regression analysis was performed with a forced entry of sex and cancer insurance coverage as covariates, and general malaise and happier now than when young (variables with $p < 0.05$ in univariate analysis) and unable to sleep (variables with $p < 0.06$ in univariate analysis). The significance level was set at 5%. SPSS version 27 (IBM Corporation; Armonk, NY, USA) was used for all statistical analyses.

3. Results

A total of 62 people were surveyed. Of these, 50 patients (80.6%) were included in the analysis, excluding seven patients who discontinued treatment on the day, three patients who did not agree to participate in the survey, and two patients who discontinued their responses.

Participants' median age (range) was 78.5 (75–86) years old. The median time since cancer diagnosis (range) was 17.5 (2–240) months. Activities of daily living responses were as follows: one respondent was independent for excretion and straightening their posture, and required being watched over for dressing; two respondents required being watched over and two required partial assistance for bathing; one participant required being watched over for eating meals; eight respondents required being watched over, six required partial assistance, and one required total assistance for going up and down the stairs; and seventeen respondents required partial assistance and thirteen required total assistance for meal preparation. Table 2 shows the treatment history by the frequency of visits, underlying diseases, and treatment method. Table 3 shows the different combinations of treatment modalities. Figure 1 shows the distribution of cancer sites.

Table 2. Participants' characteristics ($n = 50$).

Item		n	(%)
Age (median (range))	78.5 (75–86)		
Time since cancer diagnosis (median (range))	17.5 (2–240)		
Frequency of visits			
Every week		3	(6)
Every 2 weeks		19	(38)
Every 3 weeks		18	(36)
Other		10	(20)
Underlying diseases (multiple answers allowed)			
Circulatory system		30	(60)
Endocrine system		23	(46)
Urinary system		8	(16)
Motor system		7	(14)
Sensory system		6	(12)
Respiratory system		6	(12)
Others		12	(24)
Treatment history by treatment method (multiple answers allowed)			
Chemotherapy		49	(98)
Surgery		27	(54)
Radiation therapy		13	(26)

Table 3. Percentage of combinations of treatment modalities (multiple answers allowed) ($n = 50$).

Treatment Method	n	(%)
Surgery + Chemotherapy	20	(40.0)
Chemotherapy	17	(34.0)
Surgery + Chemotherapy + Radiation therapy	7	(14.0)
Chemotherapy + Radiation therapy	6	(12.0)

Of the 50 participants, 40 lived in the Noto Peninsula. Of these, ten participants lived in Kahoku, seven lived in Hakui, and six lived in Tsubata (Figure 2). The average Euclidean distance from Kanazawa Medical University Hospital to the government office in the participants' area of residence was 40.7 km, with the furthest municipality being Suzu at 100.6 km. A spider graph is shown in Figure 2.

A total of 29 (58.0%) respondents were aged between 75 and 80 years, and 21 (42.0%) were aged 80 years or older. There were 35 men (70.0%) and 15 women (30.0%).

The results of the univariate analysis are shown in Table 4. The proportion of respondents who were dissatisfied with their present life was significantly higher in seven respondents (70.0%) with general malaise ($p = 0.001$), ten respondents (47.6%) who did not think they were happier now than when they were younger ($p = 0.003$), and eight respondents (42.1%) who could not sleep ($p = 0.054$).

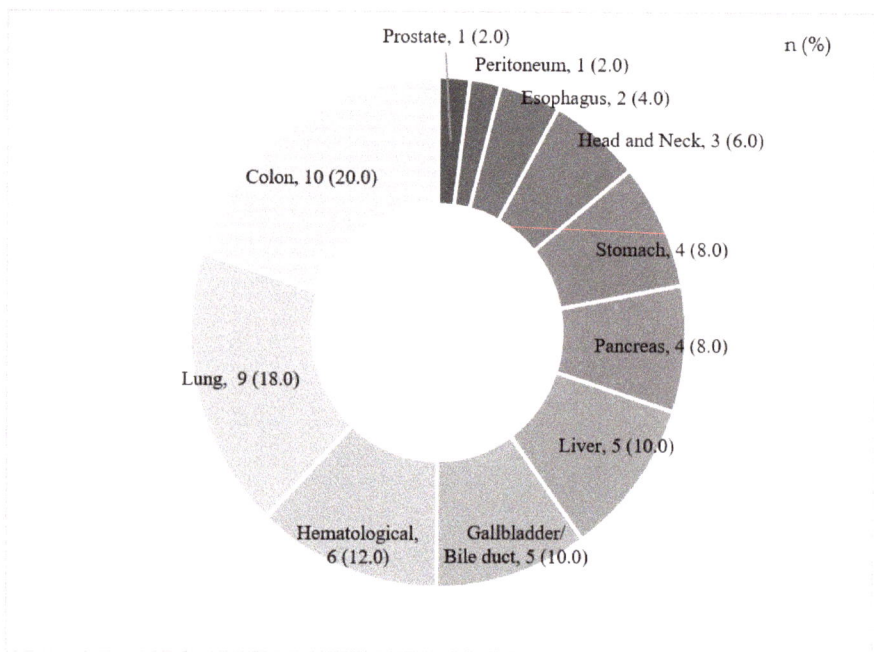

Figure 1. Cancer site (*n* = 50).

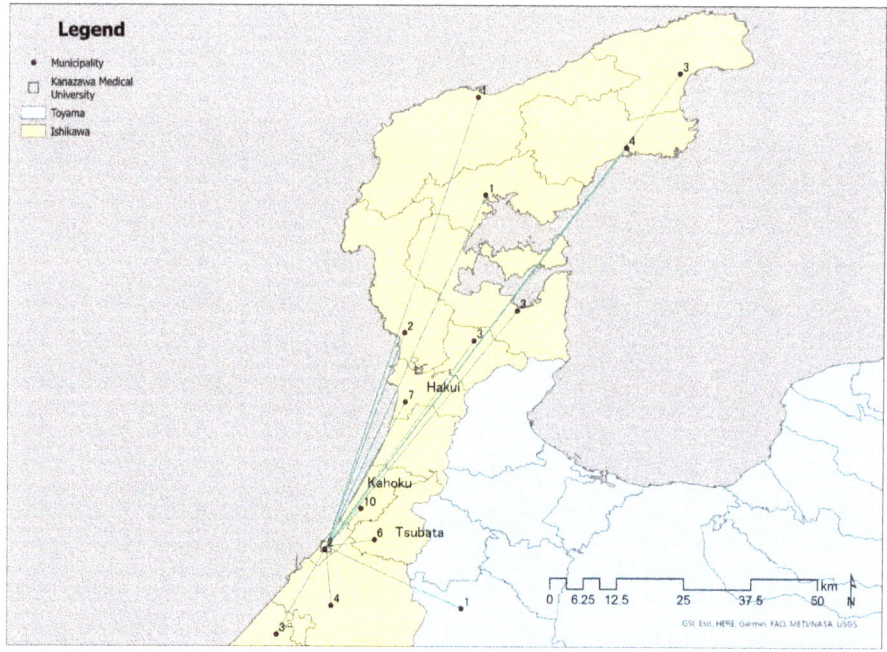

Figure 2. Spider graph.

Table 4. Association between the quality of life under treatment and current life satisfaction of cancer survivors.

Item	Category	Total N	Total %	Agree N	Agree %	Disagree N	Disagree %	p-Value
Basic attributes, annual income, cancer insurance coverage, support provider								
Age	<80	29	58.0	22	75.9	7	24.1	0.724 [a]
	≥80	21	42.0	15	71.4	6	28.6	
Sex	Male	35	70.0	24	68.6	11	31.4	0.294 [b]
	Female	15	30.0	13	86.7	2	13.3	
Annual income	2.8 million yen or above	16	32.0	11	68.8	5	31.3	0.731 [b]
	Other	34	68.0	26	76.5	8	23.5	
Cancer insurance coverage	Yes	28	56.0	21	75.0	7	25.0	0.856 [a]
	Other	22	44.0	16	72.7	6	27.3	
Co-habitants	Yes	43	86.0	33	76.7	10	23.3	0.357 [b]
	No	7	14.0	4	57.1	3	42.9	
Relatives nearby	Yes	7	14.0	4	57.1	3	42.9	0.357 [b]
	No	43	86.0	33	76.7	10	23.3	
People who would rush to help in an emergency	Yes	49	98.0	36	73.5	13	26.5	1.000 [b]
	No	1	2.0	1	100.0	0	0.0	
Time since cancer diagnosis, metastasis, underlying disease, medication status								
Time since cancer diagnosis	<17.5	25	50.0	19	76.0	6	24.0	0.747 [a]
	≥17.5	25	50.0	18	72.0	7	28.0	
Metastasis, cancer in other sites	Yes	24	48.0	19	79.2	5	20.8	0.424 [a]
	No	26	52.0	18	69.2	8	30.8	
Underlying disease	Yes	46	92.0	35	76.1	11	23.9	0.275 [b]
	No	4	8.0	2	50.0	2	50.0	
Oral medication	Yes	49	98.0	36	73.5	13	26.5	1.000 [b]
	No	1	2.0	1	100.0	0	0.0	
Opioids	Yes	1	2.0	0	0.0	1	100.0	0.260 [b]
	No	49	98.0	37	75.5	12	24.5	
Non-opioids	Yes	15	30.0	12	80.0	3	20.0	0.728 [b]
	No	35	70.0	25	71.4	10	28.6	
Cancer therapeutic drugs	Yes	13	26.0	11	84.6	2	15.4	0.469 [b]
	No	37	74.0	26	70.3	11	29.7	
Sleeping pills	Yes	6	12.0	5	83.3	1	16.7	1.000 [b]
	No	44	88.0	32	72.7	12	27.3	
Hypertension medication	Yes	21	42.0	14	66.7	7	33.3	0.314 [a]
	No	29	58.0	23	79.3	6	20.7	
Diabetes drugs	Yes	9	18.0	6	66.7	3	33.3	0.679 [b]
	No	41	82.0	31	75.6	10	24.4	
Laxatives	Yes	27	54.0	20	74.1	7	25.9	0.990 [a]
	No	23	46.0	17	73.9	6	26.1	
Physical symptoms								
General malaise	Present	10	20.0	3	30.0	7	70.0	0.001 [b]
	Other	40	80.0	34	85.0	6	15.0	
Loss of appetite	Present	15	30.0	10	66.7	5	33.3	0.493 [b]
	Other	35	70.0	27	77.1	8	22.9	
Pain	Present	14	28.0	11	78.6	3	21.4	0.734 [b]
	Other	36	72.0	26	72.2	10	27.8	
Constipation	Present	17	34.0	10	58.8	7	41.2	0.099 [b]
	Other	33	66.0	27	81.8	6	18.2	
Respiratory distress	Present	6	12.0	4	66.7	2	33.3	0.643 [b]
	Other	44	88.0	33	75.0	11	25.0	

Table 4. Cont.

Item	Category	Total		Satisfaction with Current Life				p-Value
				Agree		Disagree		
		N	%	N	%	N	%	
Other	Present	19	38.0	15	78.9	4	21.1	0.742 [b]
	Other	31	62.0	22	71.0	9	29.0	
Self-care treatment								
Being able to see a doctor at a designated date and time	Independent	45	90.0	33	73.3	12	26.7	1.000 [b]
	Other	5	10.0	4	80.0	1	20.0	
Being able to go to the hospital by oneself	Independent	25	50.0	17	68.0	8	32.0	0.333 [a]
	Other	25	50.0	20	80.0	5	20.0	
Taking oral medicines as instructed	Independent	44	88.0	32	72.7	12	27.3	1.000 [b]
	Other	6	12.0	5	83.3	1	16.7	
Satisfaction in life								
I started to worry about small things.	Agree	15	30.0	9	60.0	6	40.0	0.170 [b]
	Disagree	35	70.0	28	80.0	7	20.0	
I think I'm happier now than when I was young.	Agree	29	58.0	26	89.7	3	10.3	0.003 [a]
	Disagree	21	42.0	11	52.4	10	47.6	
I'm unable to sleep.	Agree	19	38.0	11	57.9	8	42.1	0.054 [b]
	Disagree	31	62.0	26	83.9	5	16.1	
I get agitated easily.	Agree	5	10.0	4	80.0	1	20.0	1.000 [b]
	Disagree	45	90.0	33	73.3	12	26.7	
I feel lonely.	Agree	10	20.0	5	50.0	5	50.0	0.101 [b]
	Disagree	40	80.0	32	80.0	8	20.0	
I feel uncomfortable with my family.	Agree	14	28.0	8	57.1	6	42.9	0.149 [b]
	Disagree	36	72.0	29	80.6	7	19.4	

Aged 75 Years and older receiving outpatient chemotherapy. [a] χ^2 test, [b] Fisher's exact test.

Table 5 shows the results of binary logistic regression analysis with dissatisfaction with current life as the dependent variable. In controlling for the effects of sex and cancer insurance coverage, the related factor for dissatisfaction with current life was "Yes" as opposed to "Other" for general malaise (odds ratio: 9.61; 95% confidence interval: 1.28–72.22), and "Agree" rather than "Disagree" for feeling happier now than when they were younger (odds ratio: 10.56; 95% confidence interval: 1.50–74.24) (Table 5).

Table 5. The impact of general malaise, "I think I'm happier now than when I was young", and "I'm unable to sleep" on current life satisfaction.

Item	Category	OR	95% CI		p-Value
			Lower Limit	Upper Limit	
Sex	Male/Female	2.35	0.26	21.22	0.447
Cancer insurance coverage	Yes/Other	0.92	0.11	7.44	0.938
General malaise	Yes/Others	9.61	1.28	72.22	0.028
I think I'm happier now than when I was young.	Disagree/Agree	10.56	1.50	74.24	0.018
I'm unable to sleep.	Agree/Disagree	3.16	0.53	18.92	0.208

4. Discussion

A survey of cancer patients in Japan in 2019 reported that the large intestine was the most common cancer site, followed by the lungs, stomach, and breasts [31] (Japan Cancer Information Service). According to the results for the Ishikawa Prefecture (the target area of this study) in 2016, the stomach was the most common site of cancer among registrants aged 75 and older, excluding epithelial cancer, followed by the large intestine, lungs, and colon. Issues with the digestive system were the most common symptoms in relation to cancer. Considering that the colon was also the most common site of cancer in this study, the trend seems to be similar to that among patients aged 75 years and older in Ishikawa. However, because the report indicated that cancer in the stomach, lungs, and colon (in descending order) were most common among men, and cancer in the large intestine, colon, and stomach (in descending order) were most common among women [30], lung cancer may have been ranked as second-most common in the current study because 70% of the participants were male. Kanazawa Medical University Hospital is located at the entrance of the Noto Peninsula and has been designated as a regional cancer medical care base hospital, with medical care partnerships with medical institutions on the Noto Peninsula [32] and a specialized outpatient clinic for hematology. These characteristics may have contributed to the finding that hematological cancer was the third most common cancer type in the current study. The fact that 80% of participants were patients from the Noto Peninsula may therefore be attributed to the location of the Kanazawa Medical University Hospital.

For patients receiving outpatient chemotherapy, transportation costs for those living far from treatment sites have become a major burden [33,34]. In addition, in Japan, the physical burden and fatigue of patients who must travel a long distance to visit hospitals are significant issues [35]. A study conducted in Iowa reported that patients living in areas without a chemotherapy provider had an average driving time of 58 min to receive treatment, compared with 21 min for patients living near a dedicated chemotherapy facility [36]. A study in North Carolina indicated that people who lived in rural areas more than 32 km from their chemotherapy provider were less likely to receive chemotherapy [37]. Travel distance is an important factor in outpatient cancer care in Ishikawa Prefecture, given that the study population comprised cancer survivors 75 years of age and older, the average distance of hospital visits was 40 km or more, and 80% of participants were Noto Peninsula residents. In Japan, serious accidents caused by driving errors by people aged 75 years and older have become a problem [38]. It is important to reduce the burden of hospital visits for older cancer survivors to receive chemotherapy when considering the combined symptoms of cancer, complications arising from treatment, and chemotherapy sequelae among older cancer survivors.

In Japan, 75-year-old cancer survivors have a median life expectancy of 11.9 years for men and 16.1 years for women [39]. It is important that older cancer survivors spend their remaining time satisfactorily while coping with their disease. Many cancer survivors suffer from aftereffects of cancer treatment [40]. After primary cancer treatment is completed, some symptoms continue to have a negative impact on cancer survivors for years to come. Such symptoms include physical limitations, cognitive limitations, depression, anxiety, sleep problems, fatigue, pain, and sexual dysfunction [41–43]. In particular, fatigue can persist for a long time and seriously impact QOL [44]. As previously reported, fatigue may affect life satisfaction in older cancer survivors aged 75 years and older. The response to the question of whether participants are happier now than when they were younger is a self-reported answer that involves recollection of their past condition before they had cancer. The effects of the respondents' life history and experiences (e.g., war) cannot be controlled for in comparisons between when they were younger and the present day; thus, from the current results, we cannot extrapolate a correlation between respondents thinking that they are less happy now than when they were younger and not being satisfied with their present lives. However, service providers serving older cancer survivors aged 75 years and older may be able to help survivors feel more satisfied with the rest of their lives by addressing the issues that lead them to complain that they are less happy now than when they were younger.

The current study involved several limitations. First, because we included only 50 people from one hospital, the generalizability of the study results may be limited. Second, because the current study used a self-reported survey that was conducted at an outpatient clinic, there may have been differences in the answers depending on the participant's knowledge, cognitive function, and physical condition on the day. Third, in meal preparation among activities of daily living, it was not possible to distinguish between the simple evaluation of activities and cases in which the participant does not regularly prepare meals by themselves because their spouse typically takes care of meal preparation. Finally, because this study used a cross-sectional study design, it is not possible to establish causal relationships between the variables under investigation.

5. Conclusions

In outpatient chemotherapy for older cancer survivors, it is recommended that support be provided by considering the travel distance required for treatment. As in previous studies, fatigue has been shown to impact the lives of cancer survivors aged 75 years and older. Thus, it is recommended that support providers consistently focus on the presence of fatigue while providing support.

These results suggest that some older cancer survivors with fatigue may spend the rest of their lives feeling unsatisfied with their situation. For older cancer survivors to be satisfied with their current lives, it is necessary to clarify the characteristics of fatigue they exhibit and to develop appropriate care. At present, it is recommended that support providers consistently focus on the presence of fatigue while providing support and careful observation.

Author Contributions: Conceptualization, Y.K., T.H., H.N., Y.M. (Yuko Morikawa) and Y.M. (Yoshiharu Motoo); methodology, Y.K., T.H., H.N., Y.M. (Yuko Morikawa) and Y.M. (Yoshiharu Motoo); formal analysis, Y.K. and H.N.; investigation, Y.K. and T.H.; resources, Y.K.; data curation, Y.K. and H.N.; writing (original draft preparation), Y.K. and H.N.; writing (review and editing), Y.K., H.N., Y.M. (Yuko Morikawa) and Y.M. (Yoshiharu Motoo); visualization, Y.K. and H.N.; supervision, H.N.; funding; Y.K. All authors have read and agreed to the published version of the manuscript.

Funding: This research was supported by the 35th Research Grant (2021), Hokkoku Cancer Foundation and KAKENHI JSP grant number [18K17537].

Institutional Review Board Statement: This research was conducted in accordance with the Declaration of Helsinki, 1995 (as revised in Seoul, 2008) and carried out with the consent of the university medical research ethics review committees at the authors' universities (No. I691).

Informed Consent Statement: Informed consent was obtained from all participants involved in this study.

Data Availability Statement: The data analyzed during this study are included in this published article. Further inquiries can be directed to the corresponding authors.

Acknowledgments: We thank Benjamin Knight for editing a draft of this manuscript.

Conflicts of Interest: The authors declare no conflict of interest.

References

1. Miller, K.D.; Siegel, R.L.; Lin, C.C.; Mariotto, A.B.; Kramer, J.L.; Rowland, J.H.; Stein, K.D.; Alteri, R.; Jemal, A. Cancer Treatment and Survivorship Statistics, 2016. *CA A Cancer J. Clin.* **2016**, *66*, 271–289. [CrossRef]
2. Pilleron, S.; Sarfati, D.; Janssen-Heijnen, M.; Vignat, J.; Ferlay, J.; Bray, F.; Soerjomataram, I. Global Cancer Incidence in Older Adults, 2012 and 2035: A Population-Based Study. *Int. J. Cancer* **2019**, *144*, 49–58. [CrossRef] [PubMed]
3. Bluethmann, S.M.; Mariotto, A.B.; Rowland, J.H. Anticipating the "Silver Tsunami": Prevalence Trajectories and Co-Morbidity Burden among Older Cancer Survivors in the United States. *Cancer Epidemiol. Biomark. Prev.* **2016**, *25*, 1029–1036. [CrossRef] [PubMed]
4. Parry, C.; Kent, E.E.; Mariotto, A.B.; Alfano, C.M.; Rowland, J.H. Cancer Survivors: A Booming Population. *Cancer Epidemiol. Biomark. Prev.* **2011**, *20*, 1996–2005. [CrossRef]
5. Mariotto, A.B.; Rowland, J.H.; Ries, L.A.G.; Scoppa, S.; Feuer, E.J. Multiple Cancer Prevalence: A Growing Challenge in Long-Term Survivorship. *Cancer Epidemiol. Biomark. Prev.* **2007**, *16*, 566–571. [CrossRef]
6. Pasetto, L.M.; Falci, C.; Compostella, A.; Sinigaglia, G.; Rossi, E.; Monfardini, S. Quality of Life in Elderly Cancer Patients. *Eur. J. Cancer* **2007**, *43*, 1508–1513. [CrossRef] [PubMed]
7. Thomé, B.; Hallberg, I.R. Quality of Life in Older People with Cancer–A Gender Perspective. *Eur. J. Cancer Care* **2004**, *13*, 454–463. [CrossRef]

8. Dialla, P.O.; Chu, W.-O.; Roignot, P.; Bone-Lepinoy, M.-C.; Poillot, M.-L.; Coutant, C.; Arveux, P.; Dabakuyo-Yonli, T.S. Impact of Age-Related Socio-Economic and Clinical Determinants of Quality of Life among Long-Term Breast Cancer Survivors. *Maturitas* **2015**, *81*, 362–370. [CrossRef]
9. Robb, C.; Haley, W.E.; Balducci, L.; Extermann, M.; Perkins, E.A.; Small, B.J.; Mortimer, J. Impact of Breast Cancer Survivorship on Quality of Life in Older Women. *Crit. Rev. Oncol. Hematol.* **2007**, *62*, 84–91. [CrossRef]
10. Azuero, A.; Williams, C.P.; Pisu, M.; Ingram, S.A.; Kenzik, K.M.; Williams, G.R.; Rocque, G.B. An Examination of the Relationship between Patient Satisfaction with Healthcare and Quality of Life in a Geriatric Population with Cancer in the Southeastern United States. *J. Geriatr. Oncol.* **2019**, *10*, 787–791. [CrossRef]
11. Moreno, P.I.; Ramirez, A.G.; San Miguel-Majors, S.L.; Fox, R.S.; Castillo, L.; Gallion, K.J.; Munoz, E.; Estabrook, R.; Perez, A.; Lad, T.; et al. Satisfaction with Cancer Care, Self-Efficacy, and Health-Related Quality of Life in Latino Cancer Survivors. *Cancer* **2018**, *124*, 1770–1779. [CrossRef] [PubMed]
12. Ashing, K.T.; George, M.; Jones, V. Health-Related Quality of Life and Care Satisfaction Outcomes: Informing Psychosocial Oncology Care among Latina and African-American Young Breast Cancer Survivors. *Psycho-Oncol.* **2018**, *27*, 1213–1220. [CrossRef] [PubMed]
13. Rai, A.; Han, X.; Zheng, Z.; Yabroff, K.R.; Jemal, A. Determinants and Outcomes of Satisfaction with Healthcare Provider Communication Among Cancer Survivors. *J. Natl. Compr. Cancer Netw.* **2018**, *16*, 975–984. [CrossRef] [PubMed]
14. Deimling, G.; Phelps, E.K.; Gilbert, M.; Ciaralli, S. Life Satisfaction among Older Adult, Long-Term Cancer Survivors: A Comparison of Black with White Survivors. *Psycho-Oncol.* **2019**, *28*, 1335–1341. [CrossRef]
15. Leow, K.; Lynch, M.F.; Lee, J. Social Support, Basic Psychological Needs, and Social Well-Being Among Older Cancer Survivors. *Int J. Aging Hum. Dev.* **2021**, *92*, 100–114. [CrossRef]
16. Sanda, M.G.; Dunn, R.L.; Michalski, J.; Sandler, H.M.; Northouse, L.; Hembroff, L.; Lin, X.; Greenfield, T.K.; Litwin, M.S.; Saigal, C.S.; et al. Quality of Life and Satisfaction with Outcome among Prostate-Cancer Survivors. *N. Engl. J. Med.* **2008**, *358*, 1250–1261. [CrossRef]
17. Clough-Gorr, K.M.; Ganz, P.A.; Silliman, R.A. Older Breast Cancer Survivors: Factors Associated with Change in Emotional Well-Being. *J. Clin. Oncol.* **2007**, *25*, 1334–1340. [CrossRef]
18. Dafni, U.; Tsourti, Z.; Alatsathianos, I. Breast Cancer Statistics in the European Union: Incidence and Survival across European Countries. *Breast Cancer Stat. Eur. Union* **2019**, *14*, 344–353. [CrossRef]
19. Jansen, L.; Dauphin, S.; van den Akker, M.; De Burghgraeve, T.; Schoenmakers, B.; Buntinx, F. Prevalence and Predictors of Psychosocial Problems in Informal Caregivers of Older Cancer Survivors–A Systematic Review: Still Major Gaps in Current Research. *Eur. J. Cancer Care* **2018**, *27*, e12899. [CrossRef]
20. Cabinet Office Current Status and Future Image of Aging, 2020 White Paper on Aging Society (In Japanese). Available online: https://www8.cao.go.jp/kourei/whitepaper/w-2020/html/zenbun/s1_1_1.html (accessed on 26 July 2022).
21. Ebeling, M.; Meyer, A.C.; Modig, K. The Rise in the Number of Long-Term Survivors from Different Diseases Can Slow the Increase in Life Expectancy of the Total Population. *BMC Public Health* **2020**, *20*, 1523. [CrossRef]
22. Ishikawa Prefecture Overview of Ishikawa Prefecture (In Japanese). Available online: http://www.pref.ishikawa.lg.jp/sabou/1gaiyou/index.html (accessed on 2 August 2022).
23. Ishikawa Prefecture Ishikawa Prefecture's Statistical Index (In Japanese). Available online: https://toukei.pref.ishikawa.lg.jp/search/detail.asp?d_id=4548 (accessed on 2 August 2022).
24. Ishikawa Prefecture Aging Rate in Ishikawa Prefecture (In Japanese). Available online: https://www.pref.ishikawa.lg.jp/ansin/plan/documents/zenbun2021.pdf (accessed on 14 July 2022).
25. National Cancer Center Response to Various Symptoms: National Cancer Center, Cancer Information Service: To the General Public (In Japanese). Available online: https://ganjoho.jp/public/support/condition/index.html (accessed on 2 August 2022).
26. Sainsbury, A.; Seebass, G.; Bansal, A.; Young, J.B. Reliability of the Barthel Index When Used with Older People. *Age Ageing* **2005**, *34*, 228–232. [CrossRef] [PubMed]
27. Shah, S.; Vanclay, F.; Cooper, B. Improving the Sensitivity of the Barthel Index for Stroke Rehabilitation. *J. Clin. Epidemiol.* **1989**, *42*, 703–709. [CrossRef]
28. Lawton, M.P. The Philadelphia Geriatric Center Morale Scale: A Revision1. *J. Gerontol.* **1975**, *30*, 85–89. [CrossRef] [PubMed]
29. Ranzijn, R.; Luszcz, M. Measurement of Subjective Quality of Life of Elders. *Int. J. Aging Hum. Dev.* **2000**, *50*, 263–278. [CrossRef] [PubMed]
30. Ishikawa Prefecture Cancer Registration in Ishikawa Prefecture (In Japanese). Available online: http://www.pref.ishikawa.lg.jp/kenkou/gan-touroku/top.html (accessed on 2 August 2022).
31. National Cancer Center Latest Cancer Statistics: National Cancer Center, Cancer Statistics (In Japanese). Available online: https://ganjoho.jp/reg_stat/statistics/stat/summary.html (accessed on 2 August 2022).
32. Kanazawa Medical University Hospital Regional Cancer Medical Care Base Hospital, Kanazawa Medical University Hospital, Telemedicine Support (In Japanese). Available online: http://www.kanazawa-med.ac.jp/~{}center21/cancer/gankyoten/tre/telemedicine.html (accessed on 2 August 2022).
33. Houts, P.S.; Lipton, A.; Harvey, H.A.; Martin, B.; Simmonds, M.A.; Dixon, R.H.; Longo, S.; Andrews, T.; Gordon, R.A.; Meloy, J.; et al. Nonmedical Costs to Patients and Their Families Associated with Outpatient Chemotherapy. *Cancer* **1984**, *53*, 2388–2392. [CrossRef]

34. Aviki, E.M.; Thom, B.; Braxton, K.; Chi, A.J.; Manning-Geist, B.; Chino, F.; Brown, C.L.; Abu-Rustum, N.R.; Gany, F.M. Patient-Reported Benefit from Proposed Interventions to Reduce Financial Toxicity during Cancer Treatment. *Support Care Cancer* **2022**, *30*, 2713–2721. [CrossRef]
35. Shizuoka Cancer Center. Trouble of Cancer Patients. I Am Far from the Hospital I Go to, So It Is a Burden to Go to the Hospital (In Japanese). Available online: https://www.scchr.jp/cancerqa/jyogen_3800003.html (accessed on 2 August 2022).
36. Ward, M.M.; Ullrich, F.; Matthews, K.; Rushton, G.; Tracy, R.; Bajorin, D.F.; Goldstein, M.A.; Kosty, M.P.; Bruinooge, S.S.; Hanley, A.; et al. Access to Chemotherapy Services by Availability of Local and Visiting Oncologists. *J. Oncol. Pract.* **2014**, *10*, 26–31. [CrossRef]
37. Sparling, A.S.; Song, E.; Klepin, H.D.; Foley, K.L. Is Distance to Chemotherapy an Obstacle to Adjuvant Care among the N.C. Medicaid—Enrolled Colon Cancer Patients? *J. Gastrointest. Oncol.* **2016**, *7*, 336–344. [CrossRef]
38. Cabinet Office Current Status of Traffic Accidents for the Elderly, 2017 Traffic Safety White Paper (In Japanese). Available online: https://www8.cao.go.jp/koutu/taisaku/h29kou_haku/gaiyo/features/feature01.html (accessed on 2 August 2022).
39. National Cancer Center Life Expectancy Data by Age and General Condition: National Cancer Center (In Japanese). Available online: https://ganjoho.jp/med_pro/cancer_control/medical_treatment/guideline/life_expectancy.html (accessed on 4 July 2022).
40. Ganz, P.A. Late Effects of Cancer and Its Treatment. *Semin. Oncol. Nurs.* **2001**, *17*, 241–248. [CrossRef] [PubMed]
41. Harrington, C.B.; Hansen, J.A.; Moskowitz, M.; Todd, B.L.; Feuerstein, M. It's Not over When It's Over: Long-Term Symptoms in Cancer Survivors—A Systematic Review. *Int. J. Psychiatry Med.* **2010**, *40*, 163–181. [CrossRef]
42. Ness, K.K.; Wall, M.M.; Oakes, J.M.; Robison, L.L.; Gurney, J.G. Physical Performance Limitations and Participation Restrictions Among Cancer Survivors: A Population-Based Study. *Ann. Epidemiol.* **2006**, *16*, 197–205. [CrossRef] [PubMed]
43. Mao, J.J.; Armstrong, K.; Bowman, M.A.; Xie, S.X.; Kadakia, R.; Farrar, J.T. Symptom Burden Among Cancer Survivors: Impact of Age and Comorbidity. *J. Am. Board Fam. Med.* **2007**, *20*, 434–443. [CrossRef] [PubMed]
44. Goldstein, D.; Bennett, B.; Friedlander, M.; Davenport, T.; Hickie, I.; Lloyd, A. Fatigue States after Cancer Treatment Occur Both in Association with, and Independent of, Mood Disorder: A Longitudinal Study. *BMC Cancer* **2006**, *6*, 240. [CrossRef] [PubMed]

MDPI
St. Alban-Anlage 66
4052 Basel
Switzerland
www.mdpi.com

Healthcare Editorial Office
E-mail: healthcare@mdpi.com
www.mdpi.com/journal/healthcare

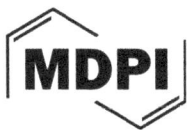

Disclaimer/Publisher's Note: The statements, opinions and data contained in all publications are solely those of the individual author(s) and contributor(s) and not of MDPI and/or the editor(s). MDPI and/or the editor(s) disclaim responsibility for any injury to people or property resulting from any ideas, methods, instructions or products referred to in the content.

www.ingramcontent.com/pod-product-compliance
Lightning Source LLC
LaVergne TN
LVHW070624100526
838202LV00012B/723